NUTRITION and YOU

with readings

William A. Forsythe III, Ph.D.
Program in Nutrition and Dietetics
School of Home Economics
University of Southern Mississippi

CPC *CONTEMPORARY PUBLISHING COMPANY*
508 ST. MARY'S STREET, RALEIGH, N.C. 27605—(919) 821-4566

PUBLISHER: Charles E. Grantham
PRODUCTION: Marianne Pair
COPYEDITING: Sheryl Fowler
TYPESETTING: Piedmont Litho
PRINTER: Edwards Brothers

ACKNOWLEDGEMENTS:
Proposed Future Food Label: Health Action Newsletter, March 1989
How's Your Diet?: Health Action Newsletter, December 1989
Calories Don't Count — Equally: Health Action Newsletter, January/February 1989
The Vitamin Pushers: Consumer Report, March 1986, pp. 170-175
How Safe is Your Food: U.S. News and World Report, November 16, 1987
Sorting Out the Cereals: Health Action Newsletter, August 1988
The Mistaken Cholesterol Myth: Health Action Newsletter, November 1989
The Right Dose: Health Action Newsletter, October 1987
Tackling High Blood Pressure: Nutrition Action Healthletter, May 1989
Are You Sure You're Getting Enough Iron?: Tufts University Diet and Nutrition Letter, October 1985 pp. 3-6
Facts and Fallacies About Eating and Pregnancy: Tufts University Diet and Nutrition Letter, December 1985
Vitamins and Minerals as Ergogenic Aids: Physician and Sport Medicine, March 1986, McGraw-Hill Publishers
Excess Proteins Leads to Osteoporosis: Health Action Newsletter, March 1987

Printed in the United States of America.

ISBN: 0-89892-083-3

TABLE OF CONTENTS

ACKNOWLEDGEMENTS

The author would like to acknowledge and thank the following persons — without whose help this book would not have been possible. Dr. Jane Boudreaux was instrumental in creating the one-credit nutrition course at the University of Southern Mississippi for which the book was written. Dr. Allison Yates secured the Department of Education (Title III) grant that provided support to write the book. She also suggested the book's title. Mr. Chuck Grantham and the editors at Contemporary Publishing provided direction and much needed editorial assistance. Finally, I am thankful for the support and encouragement of my family — my children Lara and William, and my wife Eileen.

Hattiesburg
January 1990

CHAPTER 1

Nutrition and You

Why should a student or any other person be interested in nutrition? First, everyone eats. The process of life requires that we eat to obtain the nutrients that we need to survive. Over a period of many years, scientists and researchers have elucidated the specific nutrients that are essential for life. We know that all foods are a complex mixture of thousands of chemicals. In fact, all nutrients are chemicals. A *nutrient* is a chemical that has specific functions in the body — *providing energy, providing structural components to build the body,* or *providing regulators to oversee body functions.* A basic understanding of nutrition principles will allow one to make better and more nutritious food selections.

A nutrient is a chemical that has specific functions in the body.

Another reason we should have a basic understanding of nutrition is that as our knowledge of diseases grows, it is obvious that in many instances nutrition plays a role in the development or treatment of these diseases. We know, for instance, that blood cholesterol levels can be affected by the type of fat one eats, that people with diabetes (high blood sugar) need to be concerned with the type and quantity of sugar they eat, and that a person's lifelong calcium intake can determine the strength of his bones as he becomes elderly. These are all instances of the interaction between nutrition and disease that we call health.

Individuals must take responsibility for their health. This text is titled "Nutrition and You" to emphasize that an individual can, through moderate lifestyle changes, improve his health. Good nutrition is one of the most important factors in good health.

A third reason that people should understand basic nutrition concepts is that in our society one is constantly evaluating nutritional claims. The American public is inundated with claims that it should increase this, decrease that, reduce this or change that in its diet. The public is constantly told that its food is over-processed, that its food is not natural, or that its food contains unhealthy additives or pesticides. The public receives its nutrition information from many sources: peers, advertisements, television, and so-called experts.

An uninformed public is often unable to distinguish between valid and invalid health claims. Many people believe that if something is stated on television or written in a magazine, then it must be true. But, in fact, the food product's label is the only place where claims are regulated. An understanding of nutrition will help one sort through and evaluate the money claims made about food products and supplements.

Nutrition is best gotten at the supermarket rather than the drugstore.

When one is evaluating nutrition claims, two factors need to be considered. First, any claim that sounds too good to be true is probably just that. And second, as a noted nutritionist once said, "We want people to get their nutrition from the supermarket, not the drugstore." Probably, the most basic advice for proper nutrition is simply "eat a *variety* of foods in *moderation*."

As stated previously, the foods we eat contain nutrients. We generally classify the nutrients as either macronutrients or micronutrients. The macronutrients are those nutrients consumed in large amounts. Micronutrients are those nutrients that are consumed or needed in very small quantities. Although each macronutrient and micronutrient class is covered further in separate chapters of this book, they will be introduced here.

Three of the most important macronutrients are carbohydrates, lipids and proteins.

The three most important macronutrients are *carbohydrates, lipids* (fats), and *proteins*. Carbohydrate's major function is as a dietary energy source. Dietary fats, while supplying much of the diet energy, also contribute to cell structure. Dietary proteins are used for structure and also to provide the building blocks for many regulatory proteins in the body (such as hormones and enzymes).

Micronutrients are vitamins and minerals.

The micronutrients consist of *vitamins* and *minerals. Vitamins* are *organic* compounds that regulate body processes. Nutritionists recognize thirteen vitamins: four fat-soluble and nine water-soluble vitamins. Fat-soluble vitamins are consumed with the fat portion of our foods and water-soluble vitamins are found in the watery (nonfat) part of our foods. For instance, in whole milk there is a substantial amount of vitamin A (a fat-soluble vitamin). Skim milk contains no vitamin A because in removing the fat, the vitamin A is also removed. In the United States vitamin A must, by law, be added back to the skim milk to replace that lost in processing.

Minerals are *inorganic* chemicals that, like vitamins, regulate body processes. Some of the minerals are also used as structural components (like calcium for bones and teeth). The minerals are divided, somewhat arbitrarily, into two different classes: *major minerals* and *trace elements.* There are seven major minerals found in the body in comparatively large amounts. There are fourteen different trace elements.

Recommended Daily Allowances

These thirty-seven nutrients — three macronutrients, thirteen vitamins and twenty-one minerals — are needed by the body in various quantities on a regular basis. Consumption above or below the required amounts is called *malnutrition*. Because overconsumption of nutrients is generally as bad as underconsumption, the amounts of most nutrients that individuals need to consume have been determined by the National Research Council of the National Academy of Sciences. These suggested amounts are called the *Recommended Dietary Allowances (RDA)*. Data from many experiments in both humans and animals for each nutrient are compiled, and an RDA for each nutrient is established.

Recommended Dietary Allowances are *age- and sex-adjusted*, and based on the needs of a *healthy population*. These adjustments reflect the different requirements of men and women for certain nutrients such as iron, and of both sexes at different ages in the lifecycle. These requirements are valid only for healthy people; the needs of the sick and infirm often differ from those of people in good health. Other sets of RDAs are available for pregnant or lactating (breast feeding) women.

RDAs take many factors into account.

Finally, the RDAs are *population-based*. The recommended intake of a certain nutrient is set so that the intake will meet the requirements of almost all (over 97%) of the people in whatever sex and age group one is considering. They are not absolute values for each individual in the category. Individuals are different and have different needs.

Given that the RDAs are based on general-population data, how can an individual best use this information to evaluate his dietary intake? First, he must remember that any information compiled about the nutrients in the foods he eats is only an estimate or approximation. When you evaluate your intake by keeping a record of the food you eat, rarely is the food accurately weighed. Most of the time portion size is just estimated. Plate waste is often ignored so that a person can easily over- or under-estimate the food that he is consuming.

Remember that RDAs are only estimates.

Another consideration is that when you compare the food you eat to a reference food, either using tables or nutritional analysis software, you are assuming that both foods have identical nutrient composition. Usually that is not so. You should not be overly worried if you determine that you are consuming 45 mg. of vitamin C when the RDA is 60 mg. per day. But, if one's intake is consistently less than 50% of the RDA and his food consumption for the period approximates his normal food intake pattern, then he should adjust his diet to increase consumption for that nutrient. Again, no one number should be taken as an individual's absolute requirement for a nutrient.

Four Food Groups

RDAs have been established for seventeen different nutrients. For many of the other nutrients (those for which the data is more limited or the nutrient is required in minute quantities) safe and adequate levels have been established. No one can remember each of these requirements. People consume foods not nutrients, and for the most part nutritionists would like people to think in terms of food consumption and not individual nutrients. A reasonable approach, based on concepts developed many years ago, has been used to help people think of nutrient intakes in food terms.

RDAs have been established for seventeen different nutrients.

The *four food groups* allow one a means to assess nutrient intake based on the amount and types of foods consumed (Table 1-1). The premise is that eating a variety of foods from four different groups will ensure an adequate intake of all the necessary nutrients. This system assumes that a person is consuming at least 1500 kcal from a variety of sources. If one consumes most of his calories from one food, say ice cream, even if one eats a lot of calories, the diet is too limited to get all the nutrients necessary. Conversely, even if one eats a variety of foods, unless he is eating approximately 1500 kcal, the overall intake is not sufficient to provide enough of each nutrient.

Meats and meat alternatives.

The first group is the *meats and meat alternatives group*. This group provides the protein one needs as well as energy, vitamins and minerals. One needs to eat two meat servings per day, with one serving consisting of approximately 2-3 ounces. One can consume vegetable products in place of animal meats. Two cups of soy beans or two cups of peanuts also meet a person's protein requirement.

Table 1-1. Basic four food groups.

Group	Servings/Day	Serving Portions
1. Meats	2	A. 2-3 oz. lean meat B. 3 oz. peanut butter C. 2 eggs
2. Milk	2	A. 1 cup milk B. 1-2 oz. cheese C. 2 cups ice cream
3. Cereal (Grains)	4	A. 1 slice of bread B. 1 cup of cereal
4. Fruits and Vegetables	4	A. 1 cup of greens B. 1 cup of carrots C. 1 medium orange

Milk and milk products.

The second group is the *milk and milk products group.* One needs to consume two 8-ounce glasses of milk per day to meet the requirements for this group. Substitutions are 1-2 ounces of cheese (including cottage cheese) and 2 cups of ice cream. This group primarily provides a person's daily calcium requirement. As calcium is very important in bone formation, many experts suggest that three to four servings of the milk group are necessary to optimize one's calcium intake. Pregnant or lactating women, because they have an increased calcium need, should consume four milk group servings per day. Growing children should also consume four servings of milk products per day.

Fruits and vegetables.

The third group of the basic four is the *fruits and vegetables group*. This group supplies one with many of the vitamins and minerals one needs. One should consume four different servings of fruits and vegetables each day. As previously suggested, nutritionists want people to think of their nutrient needs in terms of foods, not specific nutrients. The fruits and vegetables group provides two exceptions to this idea. One should try to eat one fruit and vegetable serving from foods rich in ascorbic acid (vitamin C) and one serving from foods rich in vitamin A. Both of these vitamins are somewhat lacking in the American diet, especially if a person does not eat a variety of foods. Good sources of ascorbic acid (vitamin C) are citrus fruits, broccoli, potatoes and strawberries. Good sources of vitamin A are dark green, leafy vegetables and orange vegetables.

The last of the basic four groups is the *cereal or grains group*. One should try to eat four servings of grains each day. A serving of grain is one slice of bread or one cup of cereal. The grains provide complex carbohydrates and many of our necessary vitamins and minerals. To increase one's intake of dietary fiber, two of the four grains servings should be whole grain such as whole wheat bread instead of white bread.

Cereal or grains.

While this classification is not foolproof, especially if one does not consume enough calories each day, this pattern of food intake does provide an easy and complete framework from which to make sound nutritional choices. For example, one could substitute a salad for a hamburger when eating at a fast food restaurant if one needed another fruits and vegetable exchange.

Nutrient Density

By most common definitions, a junk food is one that supplies "empty" calories — calories without many nutrients. Soft drinks, potato chips, candy bars and cookies are examples of so-called junk foods. However, many foods labeled as junk foods supply much more than calories even if they are not considered traditional sources of nutrients. Also, some people need calories, just as some people need to limit calories. Foods that supply just calories are not inherently bad. It is the overeating of these foods, precluding or limiting the intake of more nutritionally valuable foods, that can create problems. Within the framework of sound nutritional practices, the consumption of these so-called junk foods is, and should be, permitted. Therefore, the term junk food is considered by most nutritionists to be inappropriate. All foods supply some nutrients, albeit in sometimes limited amounts.

Junk foods are not always bad.

What should be considered in choosing foods is their *nutrient density*. Nutrient density is a concept that evaluates foods on the basis of the nutrients per kilocalorie. In the United States we generally eat foods that are not very nutrient-dense; many of the processed foods that we consume contain a lot of kilocalories but not as many nutrients (vitamins and minerals) as we need. Within the framework of a sound diet, one should not feel guilty about eating a candy bar, cola drink or potato chips. But one should be aware that these foods are not providing very many nutrients except for fats and sugar. By thinking in terms of nutrient density and the basic four food groups, it is possible to partake of a diet that contains all of the nutrients one would need.

A good example illustrating the principle of nutrient density is found in the milk group. Milk and other milk-group products are the major source of dietary calcium. A glass of milk, while containing about 250 mg of calcium, also provides about 160 kilocalories. A glass of skim milk, containing approximately the same amount of calcium, only contains about 80 kcal. Thus, skim milk is more nutrient-dense than whole milk; while both provide the same amount of calcium, skim milk does so with less kilocalories. To consume the same amount of calcium as in a glass of whole milk, you need to consume about 320 kcal of ice cream. Cheese is also less nutrient-dense than whole milk. To get an equivalent amount of calcium, one must consume 250 kcal of cheese. Using the concept of nutrient density, a person can try to substitute more nutrient-dense foods for less nutrient-dense foods.

Food and Nutritional Labels

Most people are unaware of the substantial information that must be present on a food label. In the following section the information required on food packages will be discussed.

While we assume that a food label will include the food product's name, it was only in 1967 that a law was passed — "The Truth in Labeling Law" — that standardized the way this information is presented. The *product name* must be prominently displayed on the

Table 1-2. Food Labeling Claims

WELL DEFINED TERMS — (as defined by the Food and Drug Administration)

1. **Low Calorie:** no more than 40 kcals per serving and no more than 0.4 kcals per gram.
2. **Reduced Calorie:** one-third fewer kcals than the original product.
3. **Sugar-free/sugarless:** can mean either:
   a. contains no carbohydrate sweeteners (sucrose, fructose, corn syrup or honey) **and** is low or reduced in kcals.
   b. contains sugar alcohols (sorbitol or xylitol). These sugars contain the same number of kcals as regular sugar but the product has a specific purpose (i.e., used by diabetics, or used to control tooth decay).
4. **Products advertising less fat:**
   a. **Lean:** not more than 10 percent fat by weight.
   b. **Extra Lean:** not more than 5 percent fat by weight.
   c. **Leaner:** at least 25 percent less fat, by weight than the regular product.
5. **Salt Advertising:**
   a. **Sodium-free:** no more than 5 mg sodium per serving.
   b. **Very Low Sodium:** no more than 35 mg sodium per serving.
   c. **Low Sodium:** no more than 140 mg sodium per serving.
   d. **No salt added:** no salt added during processing. Food could have high amounts of salt naturally, or sodium could be present from other ingredients in product.
6. **Cholesterol Claims:**
   a. **Cholesterol-free:** less than 2 mg cholesterol per serving.
   b. **Low Cholesterol:** less than 20 mg cholesterol per serving.
   c. **Reduced Cholesterol:** must have 75 percent less cholesterol than original product.

CONTROVERSIAL TERMS — (these terms have no legal definition)

1. **Natural:** Not defined legally.
2. **Organic:** Implies no synthetic fertilizers or pesticides were used in growing the product. But organic has no legal definition and it is impossible to know how a product was grown.
3. **No Sugar Added:** Suggests that a product is unsweetened. Some products (cereals, granola bars) may claim "no sugar added" but may add concentrated fruit juices (a source of sugars).
4. **Lite/Light:** Can denote a food that is lower in salt, sugar, kilocalories, alcohol, fat or even lighter in color than a similar product. You must read the label carefully to find out why the product is designated light. Lite Potato Chips may only refer to their color.

1. Adapted from: *On Your Mark.* The Sugar Association 1101-15th Street, Washington, D.C. May, 1989.

package in *bold letters*. This name must accurately represent the product make-up. For instance, a product called "Corn and Peas" must have more corn than peas. A question is always raised about "Pork and Beans," because there are usually more beans than pork in these products. A few traditional products such as "Pork and Beans" were allowed to keep their names. If the product uses artificial flavors, this must also be prominently displayed near the product name, such as "Vanilla Pudding with artificial flavor."

In addition to the product name, a food package must always display the *manufacturer's name and address*. The *net weight* (weight without the package) must also be displayed.

Another part of this law states that food packages must not deceive the consumer regarding the amount of the product contained in the package. Food packages must be at least ninety percent full. Exceptions to this rule include potato chips and cereal. These products tend to settle, not completely filling the package. As you have probably noticed, these products must carry a disclaimer stating that: "the contents of this package are sold by weight. Some settling may occur during shipping."

Health and nutritional claims are appearing more often on food package labels. The Food and Drug Administration (FDA) regulates these claims. The FDA's current position on health claims (i.e., "oat bran will lower your cholesterol") is that the claim can only be used if it represents a "significant scientific consensus." Nutritional claims are harder to regulate. Table 1-2 provides examples of nutritional claims one might find on a food label.

Ingredient labels provide valuable information.

The *ingredient label* is another part of the food package. Ingredient labels tell the consumer what is in the food product. The ingredients must be listed in descending order of predominance in the food product. Thus, the first item listed on an ingredient label is the product's primary ingredient. The ingredients list on a can of "Pork and Beans" might read as follows: beans, water, pork, and salt. This would mean that while there are more beans than pork, there is also more water than pork in the product. Probably in the near future, the amount of each ingredient will be specified in the ingredient list. The ingredient label for "Pork and Beans" might then look as follows: beans (63%), water (28%), pork (8%), and salt (1%).

Products that have a *standard of identity* are not required by law to display an ingredients list. Standards of identity for products were developed in the 1930s to bring consistency to food products. The public knew that any product covered by a standard of identity had similar ingredients. Many products, including bread, pasta, salad dressing and mayonnaise, ice cream, ketchup and tomato paste, have standards of identity. This means that any product that calls itself mayonnaise must contain certain ingredients in certain specified amounts. If the product is not made as the recipe of the standard of identity for mayonnaise dictates, then that product must be clearly labeled imitation mayonnaise. Currently, most products that are covered by standards of identity also list the ingredients on the label. Nowadays the consumer is more inclined to buy a product that lists its ingredients than one that does not, so it is to the manufacturer's advantage to list ingredients.

Nutritional labels

A final component of the food label is the *nutritional label* (Table 1-3). By law, a food must display a nutritional label if: 1) the food makes a nutritional claim (i.e., low-salt, high-calcium, etc.); 2) adds a nutrient (i.e., iron-fortified cereals, Hi-C drinks, etc.); or 3) the food makes dietary claims (i.e., low-calorie). About one-third of our foods are required by law to carry a nutritional label. However, over 70% of the foods on the supermarket shelf carry nutritional labels, so manufacturers must believe they are popular.

Serving size

One can divide the nutritional label into three components. The first component is the serving size (Table 1-3A). The servings-per-container are usually listed at the top of the nutritional label. One serving is what all the values are based upon. For most foods, "one serving" represents a serving for the average adult man.

Macronutrients

The second area (Table 1-3B) of the nutritional label contains information about the macronutrients (protein, fat and carbohydrate) and kilocalories in the product. If a product makes a claim about its cholesterol or fat content, then this information must also be placed in this section of the label. Products that make claims about the kind of carbohydrates (simple sugars versus complex carbohydrates) or the amount of dietary fiber the product contains must also provide this specific information on the nutritional label. A recent law requires that the amount of sodium (in mg) in a product also be listed in this section.

Table 1-3. Example of nutritional label for canned green beans.

Nutrition Information

A Servings Size = 1 cup; Servings per container = 2

B		
	Calories	125
	Protein	6 g
	Carbohydrate	23 g
	Fat	2 g
	Sodium	180 mg

Percentage of U.S. Recommended Daily Allowance (U.S. RDA)

C				
	Protein	10	Niacin	15
	Vitamin A	25	Calcium	6
	Vitamin C	20	Iron	4
	Thiamin	8	Vitamin B_6	*
	Riboflavin	*	Vitamin B_{12}	*

*Product contains less than 2% of the U.S. RDA for these nutrients.

The third section of the nutritional label (Table 1-3C) provides information about how well a serving of the product meets the U.S. RDA for nutrients. The U.S. RDA is very similar to the RDA except that men and women are grouped together, with the RDA that is highest for either sex being the U.S. RDA. For instance, the RDA for iron is 10 mg/day for men and 18 mg/day for women. In this case, the U.S. RDA would be 18 mg/day. In the following nutritional label example, the canned green beans would provide 4% of the needed 18 mg. If a product is not a very good source of a nutrient, containing less than 2%, an asterisk may be used in place of a value for that nutrient. The statement "this product contains less than 2% of the U.S. RDA for this nutrient" follows this section.

RDA requirements

By law, information on the U.S. RDAs for protein and the nine nutrients listed in the example must be presented on the nutritional label. Information on an additional 10 nutrients may voluntarily be included. Usually, if a product is a poor source of potassium or zinc, the manufacturer will not include this information on the label. However, if the product is a good source of a nutrient, the manufacturer will usually add this information to the label.

Must nutritionists believe that nutritional labels are too complex. Too much information and too many nutrients are required to be listed. Remember, one should eat foods, not nutrients. In the future labels will be much simpler. One suggestion is that only information for vitamin A, vitamin C, calcium, and iron be required in the U.S. RDA section. An example of a proposed food label is shown in Table 1-4.

Although food and nutrition labels contain valuable information about food products, this information should only complement basic nutrition practice. While the following chapters provide information about specific nutrients, all a person really needs to remember is to eat a variety of foods from the basic four food groups and to eat those foods in moderation. It is not necessary to exist on exotic diets to be healthy. Nor is it necessary to feel guilty if one doesn't always eat the most healthful foods. Just try for variety and moderation!

Table 1-4. An example of a proposed future food label.
(*Nutrition Action Healthletter*. Center for Science in the Public Interest, Vol. 16. March, 1989).

PERCENT OF CALORIES:
The pie chart breaks down a single serving of the product, and shows what percent of its calories comes from each major nutrient.

This Macaroni & Cheese doesn't look too good. It gets nearly half its calories from fat, which is well above the American Heart Association's goal of 30 percent for the overall diet. In addition, 20 percent of the product's calories comes from "cholesterol-raising" fat. That's about twice as much as is generally recommended.

IMPORTANT INFORMATION:
All the product's vital statistics are listed. That means information on fiber, cholesterol, cholesterol-raising fat, sodium, carbohydrates, protein, calcium, iron, and vitamins A and C.

OILS: *No more anonymous oils. Each oil used must be named. (Quaker lists the oil content of its Caramel Nut Granola Dipps as "coconut oil and/or palm kernel oil and/or palm oil and/or soybean oil and/or cottonseed oil.")*

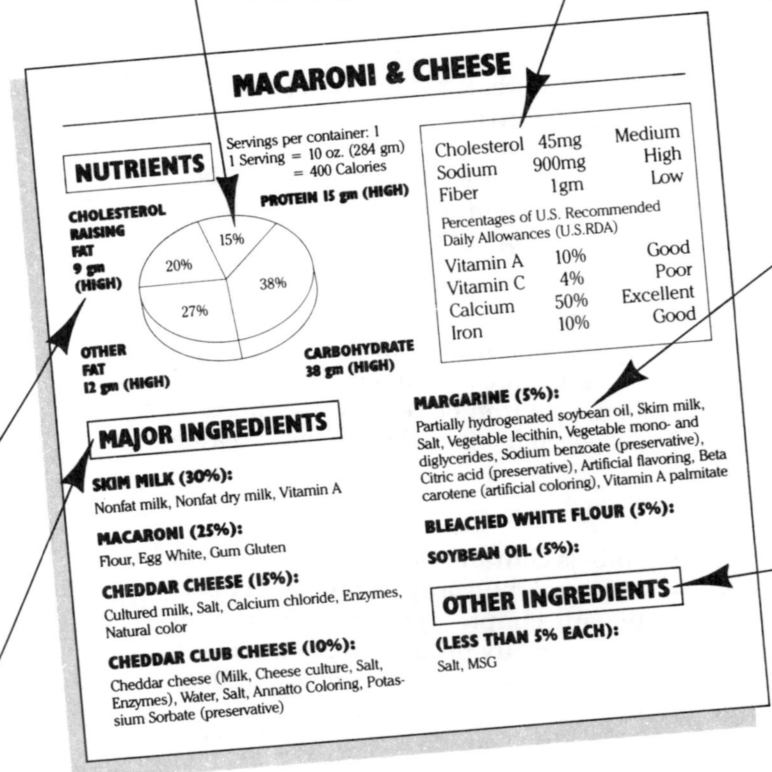

Here's how the same macaroni & cheese product might look *if we were designing its label.*

FAT BREAKDOWN:
"Cholesterol-raising" fat includes all saturated fats except stearic acid, which doesn't seem to elevate cholesterol levels. (The fats that comprise each group would change as new evidence emerges.)

OTHER INGREDIENTS:
Ingredients making up less than five percent of the product (by weight) are listed separately. The listing of all synthetic dyes (not just Yellow No. 5) is mandatory.

MAJOR INGREDIENTS:
Ingredients that make up five percent or more of the product's weight are listed in descending order. Each ingredient's percent is given, which makes it easy to see if we're paying macaroni & cheese prices for something that's 30 percent skim milk.

If the product contains sugars, they'll have to drop all their disguises (caramel, corn syrup, dextrose, high fructose corn sweetener, honey, malt, etc.) and be grouped together as one ingredient.

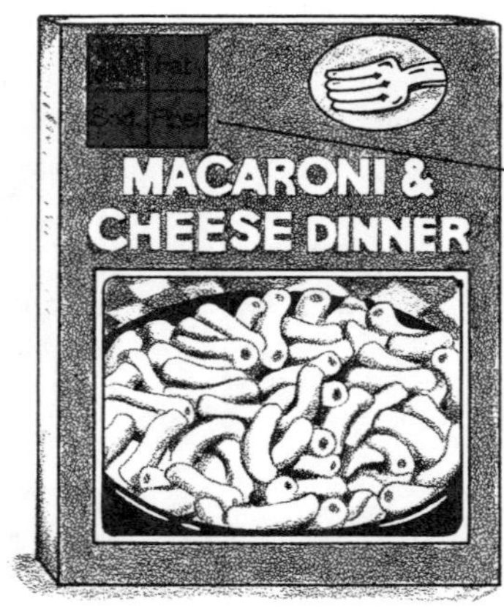

STOPLIGHTS: *The front of the package has a box with four "stoplights." Each tells consumers if the product is high or low in an important nutrient.*

The "sodium," "fat," and "fiber" stoplights are shaded red, which means the Macaroni & Cheese is high in the baddies (sodium and fat) and low in the goodie (fiber). Since the number of calories is moderate, the "calorie" stoplight is yellow. If the product were high in a good nutrient or low in a bad one, that nutrient's stoplight would be green.

ILLUSTRATION: LOEL BARR

MARCH 1989

HORIZONS

A *U.S. News* test helps resolve cancer questions about pesticides

How safe is your food?

■ "A grim specter has crept upon us almost unnoticed." Thus did naturalist Rachel Carson's landmark work, *Silent Spring,* awaken the public to the profligate use of DDT and other pesticides. But 25 years later, her legacy is a tripling of pesticide volume—390,000 tons a year in the U.S., or more than 3 pounds for each person. No wonder 3 out of 4 people surveyed last February by the Food Marketing Institute, a trade group representing supermarket chains, consider pesticides and herbicides to be a "serious health hazard." And in a telephone survey in July by the Alliance for Food and Fiber, an organization representing California food growers, 45 percent of Californians disapproved of farmers' using pesticides.

Sheer chemical tonnage and public concern notwithstanding, most scientists believe the cancer threat from pesticides in food is minuscule next to smoking and other known causes. A sizable minority even believes that the threat pales beside the cancer risk posed by the chloroform in ordinary tap water and by natural substances in foods. But there are enough gaps—and occasionally chasms—in what is known about pesticides that scientists often clash over just how stringent pesticide regulations need to be.

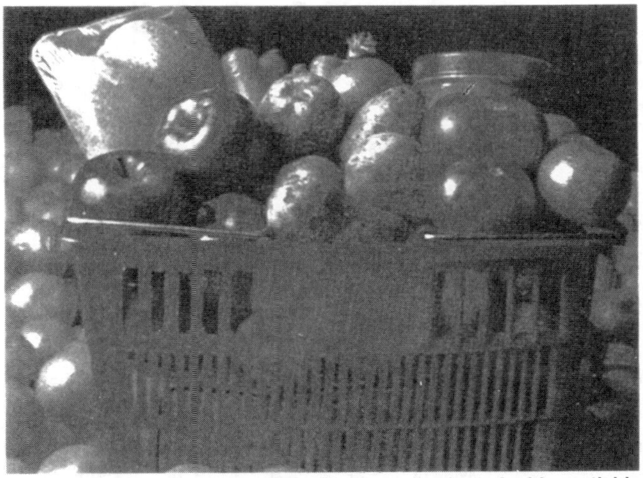

CHARLIE ARCHAMBAULT FOR USN&WR

Is this collection of ordinary food items contaminated with pesticide residues? We put just such a market-basket assortment to the test

Looking for residues

One key question is, just how much pesticide remains on food by the time it gets to the supermarket? Based on government and industry tests, the answer is, very little. If true, that's reassuring. To check this premise and to see whether residues of common pesticides are likely to exceed current legal limits, *U.S. News* commissioned an ambitious test. Last August, the month when growers' use of pesticides normally peaks, couriers collected samples of seven raw foods and two types of processed foods from wholesale markets in New York City, St. Louis and San Francisco. The foods, unwashed, were shipped within 24 hours to the National Food Laboratory, a Dublin, Calif., firm well known for its food research and testing. Each food item was checked for a carcinogenic pesticide commonly used on that food. The study was designed with the help of the Center for Investigative Reporting, a nonprofit group in San Francisco with extensive experience in pesticide research. Full results appear on the facing page.

What's most significant about the results, even though they are too limited to justify broad conclusions, is what they do not show: Of 87 tests for specific chemicals, 82 turned up nothing at all. In all five cases that tested positive, the pesticide residue was less than one fourth of the amount that is permitted by law. An orange from San Francisco's wholesale market registered the highest cancer hazard, containing 2.6 parts per million of benomyl, one of the most common fungicides used in agriculture. According to a worst-case estimate based on Environmental Protection Agency figures, if every orange eaten over a lifetime contains at least that amount of benomyl, there would be 1 additional cancer in every 166,000 people. Compare that with the 1 chance in 5,400 of dying in a car crash in the United States.

But how good are the EPA numbers? The way scientists assess the cancer hazard of any substance is to feed high doses of it to laboratory animals. If any dosage causes tumors in any species tested, the substance is labeled a carcinogen. By this definition, at least 53 of about 300 pesticides used on food crops in the United States are carcinogenic. Mathematical models turn the findings into numerical risk estimates. A pesticide considered a potent carcinogen might cause 1 additional case of cancer for every 10,000 people. An extremely weak carcinogen may carry a risk of 1 additional cancer in 1 billion people.

It sounds straightforward. But the assumptions that underlie such risk assessments are widely challenged. Many scientists question whether chemicals that cause cancers at high dosages in animals pose any hazard in the trace amounts in typical diets.

How tolerant?

In shaping public policy, caution is customary. The EPA limits pesticides' residues to specified amounts. The limit is called a tolerance. The more potent the carcinogen, the lower the tolerance level.

At least, that's how it is supposed to work. But as a blue-ribbon panel at the National Academy of Sciences (NAS) reported last May, the EPA's standards are glaringly inconsistent. Its regulations hold new pesticides to very high—even impossible—standards, yet permit older, more worrisome pesticides to stay on the market. Most of these pesticides were approved before 1978, when the agency began to demand more-stringent health data. Today, 10 of these older chemicals are still widely used in agriculture—and account for as much as 90 percent of our dietary cancer risk. What's more, they are extremely difficult to detect. Says Richard Wiles, staff director of the NAS panel: "The government has only a crude idea how much of these pesticides are being served up on our plates."

To better protect public health, the NAS report recommended that the EPA scrap its crazy-quilt rules and instead apply a "negligible risk" standard to all pesticides across the board. As the report defined it, a negligible risk would cause no more than 1 additional case of cancer in every million people exposed to the pesticide in their diet over a 70-year lifetime.

How do the pesticides in the *U.S. News* study square up in the light of the proposed standard? All were approved before 1978, and three of the five residues that passed the current EPA standards would have flunked the NAS negligible-risk standard. Moreover, a fourth residue just squeaks by.

Several consumer groups feel that even the NAS recommendations don't go far enough. The main worries of these groups center on what we don't know. Ellen Haas, executive director of Public Voice for Food and Health Policy, is alarmed by what she calls "an astounding dearth of adequate health data." Although somewhat exaggerated, her point does have validity: About three dozen pesticides have never been tested in animal-cancer studies. The EPA says that many of them are obsolete or seldom used, but it can't furnish a precise number. The question of pesticide combinations also remains open. A 1984 study by the National Resources Defense Council found that 42 percent of pesticide-tainted food samples had been treated with more than one pesticide.

Repellent carcinogens

Many scientists disagree with the position of the NAS and the consumer groups, however. These scientists are led by Bruce Ames, the biochemist who developed today's most widely used test for identifying potential cancer-causing substances. In their view, the present regulations go quite far enough because, says Ames, "the dietary dose is so small as to pose a trivial risk."

Ames and his followers argue that most common foods contain large amounts of natural substances at levels hundreds or even thousands of times more carcinogenic than residues of the most dangerous pesticides concocted by the chemical industry. Fruits and vegetables apparently produce these substances for the purpose of repelling insects, fungi and other predators—a surprise that came to light when scientists began to test natural-food constituents under the same guidelines that regulatory agencies use to identify man-made carcinogens.

Suppose that before the potent carcinogen EDB was banned, you consumed traces of the pesticide in your food in an amount typical of most U.S. adults. By Ames's calculations, a daily glass of wine is 10,000 times more likely to give you cancer than is ingesting residues of EDB—and 1,000 times more dangerous than the leftover residues of Rachel Carson's hated DDT. The natural cancer-causing agents in 1 leaf of basil, 1 teaspoon of brown mustard or even a single raw mushroom are hundreds or thousands of times more carcinogenic than residues of DDT and EDB.

Ames doesn't want to kill your appetite. He doubts that even natural carcinogens are concentrated enough in the normal diet to cause harm. Rather, he wants hazards put in perspective. Says Ames: "Just remember you're consuming 10,000 times more of Mother Nature's pesticides."

Potato chemistry

The NAS panelists think Ames's arguments make sense—but feel they can't afford to treat pesticide risks casually. Clearly, diet *can* have a big impact on cancer. In Japan, for example, there's abundant stomach cancer but relatively little breast cancer. When Japanese immigrate to the U.S. and adopt a Western diet, however, their likelihood of developing these cancers reverses, becoming the same as for the rest of the U.S. population. But isolating the responsible substance, or substances, is devilishly hard. A potato alone contains 150 chemicals—before it's doused with pesticides.

Given the unknowns, the NAS panel chose to act conservatively. Says panel member Dr. Arthur Upton, a New York University cancer specialist: "We haven't lived with many [man-made] pesticides long enough to say with certainty that they pose a trivial risk."

There are other reasons for regulating pesticides apart from the food-safety issue. Even Ames believes farmers may inhale dangerous amounts of pesticides or absorb chemicals through their skin. Worse, pesticides are being detected in the ground water in intensively farmed areas, exposing farmers and nearby populations to additional hazards through their drinking water. The concentrations are usually too low to pose any threat, but the situation is sure to worsen. Pesticides break down slowly beneath the ground, where there are few bacteria and no sunlight.

The EPA is expected to enact the panel's recommendations as early as next January. Meanwhile, if you're concerned about carrying chemicals home with your tomatoes, consumer groups advise washing fruits and vegetables with soapy water. Ames simply suggests a varied diet, so that no one chemical—whether natural or created in a lab—overwhelms your body's defenses. Perhaps most important, keep the threat in perspective. If you smoke cigarettes or drink alcohol, concerns about chemicals in our food should be taken with a grain of salt. ■

by Kathleen McAuliffe with David Gilbert, William Kistner and David Weir from the Center for Investigative Reporting in San Francisco

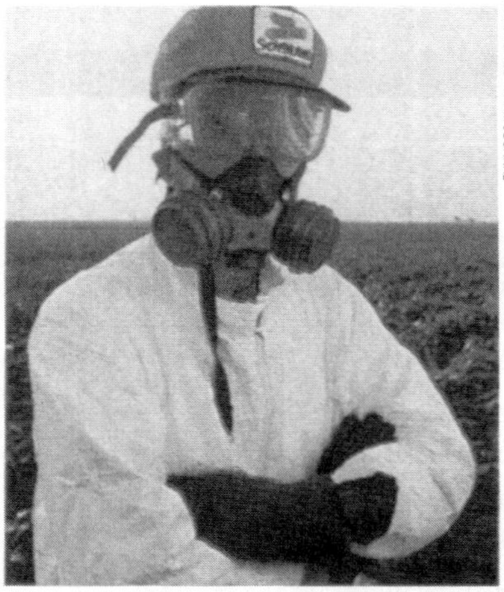

DAVE TONGE—FARM JOURNAL

Illinois farmer Dan Chambers, equipped to spray pesticides on his crops

LIFE'S HAZARDS

Are pesticides the problem?

The pesticides DDT and EDB are such potent cancer threats that they've been banned. Yet their cancer-causing potential, compared with that of ordinary city tap water and a variety of common foods, is believed to be tiny. The reason: Naturally occurring chemicals in these foods—the estragole in dried basil and the aflatoxin in peanut butter, for example—are much more carcinogenic than pesticides, because we consume them in far greater amounts. The ranking system below, comparing the cancer risk from DDT and EDB with that of eight substances found in many people's diets, was conceived by biochemist Bruce Ames of the University of California at Berkeley and Renae Magaw and Lois Swirsky Gold of the Lawrence Berkeley Laboratory. The hazards are based on a typical person's average daily exposure to the substance over a lifetime and are calculated as a percentage of the dose that causes cancer in half of exposed rodents. Hence the name of the numerical index: HERP, for Human Exposure Dose/Rodent Potency.

Cancer hazard	Food *(carcinogen)*
.0003	DDT, from residues remaining
.0004	EDB, before ban took effect
.001	Municipal tap water, 4 8-oz. glasses *(chloroform)*
.03	Peanut butter, 1 sandwich *(aflatoxin)*
.03	Comfrey tea, 1 cup *(symphytine)*
.07	Brown mustard, 1 teaspoon *(allyl isothiocyanate)*
.1	Dried basil, 1 leaf *(estragole)*
.1	Raw mushrooms, 1 *(hydrazines)*
2.8	Beer, 12-oz. bottle *(ethyl alcohol)*
4.7	Wine, 8-oz. glass *(ethyl alcohol)*

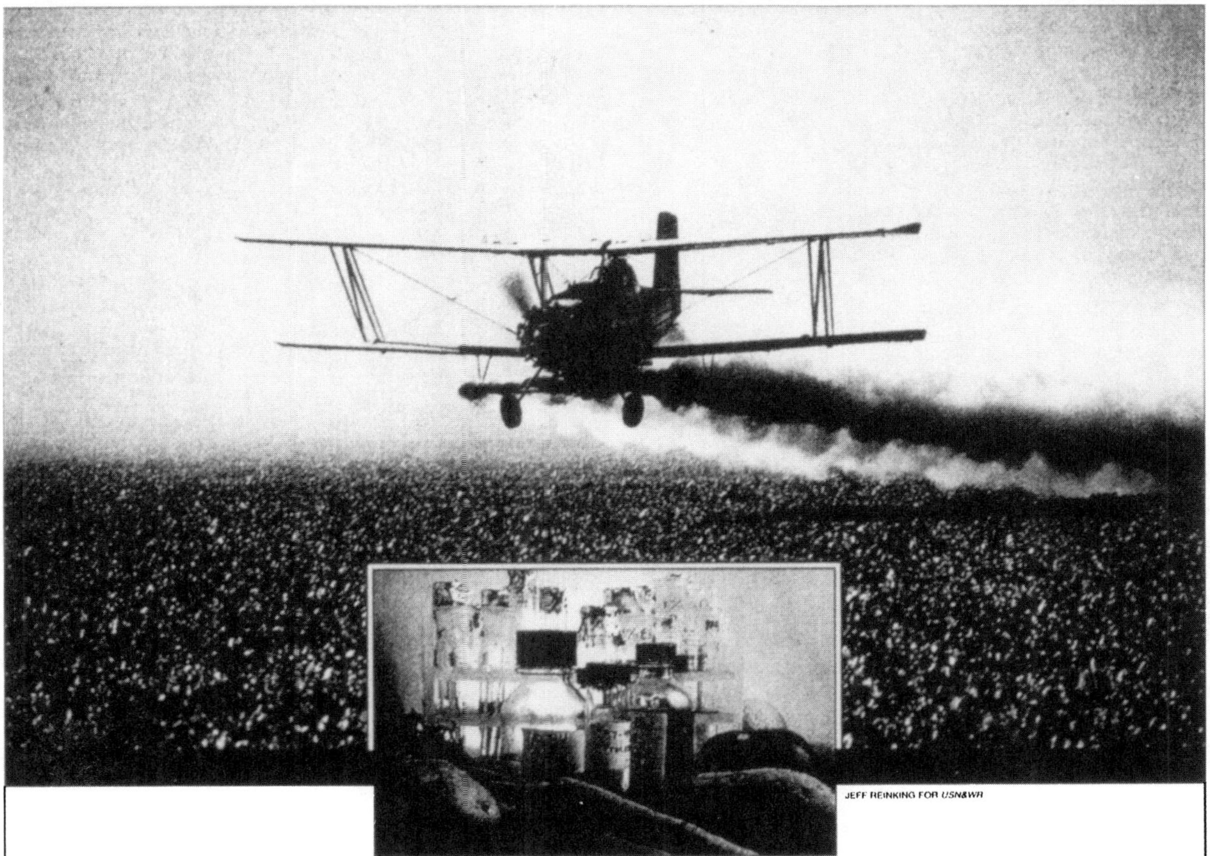

JEFF REINKING FOR *USN&WR*

The raw materials and tools of food testing

U.S.News & WORLD REPORT

LEGALLY CLEAN, BUT QUESTIONS REMAIN

In the *U.S. News* test, two samples of eight different foods were collected in each of three cities. In addition, one sample of peanut butter was collected in each city. The 51 samples underwent 87 tests for pesticides. Five of the 51 samples showed some evidence of pesticide residues. All five easily passed legal limits now in effect, but three of the five would fail a negligible-risk standard that has been proposed by the National Academy of Sciences.

	Pesticide checked	Samples containing pesticide	Source of tainted food	Residue as proportion of legal limit	Meets proposed NAS risk standard
Oranges	Benomyl	1 of 6	San Francisco	1/4	No (1 in 166,000)
Apples	Daminozide	0 of 6		None	
	Maneb	1 of 6	New York	1/4	No (1 in 235,000)
Peaches	Benomyl	1 of 6	New York	1/100	Yes (1 in 14 mil.)
Strawberries	Folpet	1 of 6	New York	1/33	Yes (1 in 1 mil.)
	Organophosphates	0 of 6		None	
Peanut butter	Daminozide	1 of 3	St. Louis	1/30	No (1 in 303,000)
Tomatoes	EBDC's	0 of 6		None	
	ETU	0 of 6		None	
	Organophosphates	0 of 6		None	
Tomato paste	EBDC's	0 of 6		None	
	ETU	0 of 6		None	
Potatoes	EBDC's	0 of 6		None	
	ETU	0 of 6		None	
Carrots	Chlorinated hydrocarbons	0 of 6		None	

Note: Proposed National Academy of Sciences risk standard would ban pesticides judged to cause more than 1 case of dietary cancer for every 1 million people. Orange had 2.6 parts per million of benomyl; legal maximum, 10 ppm. Apple had 0.5 ppm of maneb; legal maximum, 2 ppm. Peach had 0.14 ppm of benomyl; legal maximum, 15 ppm. Strawberry had 0.76 ppm of folpet; legal maximum, 25 ppm. Peanut butter had 1 ppm of daminozide; legal maximum, 30 ppm.

Name ______________________

Section ______________________

Date ______________________

Chapter 1

QUESTIONS FOR REVIEW

1. List three functions of a nutrient.

   a. dev - growth

   b. reprod

   c. maintance

2. Consumption of nutrients above or below required levels is called malnutrition.

3. Recommended Daily Allowances (RDAs) are suggested intake levels of nutrients for healthy people. RDAs are also age and sex-adjusted and population-based.

4. List the four food groups and the suggested daily servings of each group.

Group	Servings per day
a. cereal/grain	4 (6-11)
b. milk	4 (2-3)
c. veg/fruit	4 (3-5)
d. meat	2 (2-3)

5. Foods that have a lot of nutrients per kilocalorie are said to be nutrient density.

6. List the three items that must be on every food label.

   a. name (prod)

   b. net wt.

   c. manuf. name + address

7. When must a food have a nutritional label?

   a. nutritional claim

   b. dietary food (lite)

CHAPTER 2

Nutritional Assessment and Energy Metabolism

Before making dietary recommendations to someone, it is important to know the health and nutritional status of that person. Nutritional assessments of an individual take many forms (Table 2-1).

Table 2-1. Nutritional assessment categories.

1. Personal Histories
   A. Medical
   B. Drug
   C. Diet
2. Physical Measurements (anthropometric measurements)
   A. Weight
   B. Height
   C. Skinfold thicknesses
3. Laboratory Measurements
   A. Blood pressure
   B. Blood cholesterol levels
   C. Blood glucose levels

Personal Histories: Before nutrition information can be given to a person, it is necessary to know something of his medical history. Many medical problems such as diabetes, hypertension, kidney problems, and heart disease affect nutritional status. A person's drug history is also important because many prescription drugs interfere with nutrient absorption, metabolism and excretion. The average elderly person takes 3 to 8 prescription medicines per day. Many antibiotics such as penicillin interfere with the absorption of certain vitamins. A person may have an adequate intake of a nutrient, but because of interactions with a prescription drug, he may still develop symptoms of deficiency of that nutrient. For such reasons, one can fully evaluate someone's nutritional status only by knowing the complete medical history of that person.

Medical and drug histories must be taken into consideration.

Diet Histories: A nutritional assessment would not be complete without a *diet history*. Diet histories take three forms: 24-hour recall, 3-day food diary, and food-frequency survey. Each method has advantages and disadvantages over the other methods. However, if properly done, each method will provide a reliable indication of the food consumption patterns of an individual.

Diet history is also important.

The 24-hour recall

The *24-hour recall survey* is the easiest dietary survey to conduct. In this survey, a person writes down all the foods and the approximate quantities consumed over the last 24 hours. Then the foods and amounts eaten are entered into a nutritional analysis program on a computer to generate individual nutrient intake. The major advantage of the 24-hour recall over other food assessment methods is that this technique is fast and easy to do at any time during an office visit. Either the subject can work on his own, or sometimes a nutritionist will work with the subject to recall the foods eaten over the past 24 hours. Nutritionists conducting food-recalls will often use food models (plastic or rubber representations of foods). The use of food models provides the subject with visual clues and also allows better estimates of the quantity of a food consumed by the person. Each model generally represents a common portion size for that food. So the interviewer can ask, "Did you eat more of this product, or less?"

One major problem with the 24-hour recall is that often, even when prompted, people just do not (sometimes on purpose) remember all the foods they ate during the previous 24 hours. This is especially true with obese subjects. So, 24-hour recall surveys often underestimate the total food consumption of a person.

Another drawback of the 24-hour recall method is that the food eaten over the last 24 hours by a person, even if he perfectly remembers all of it, may not represent the usual intake pattern of that individual. This is especially true of 24-hour recalls conducted on Mondays; the food eaten on Sunday is often very different for most people than the food eaten during the week. Even given the limitations, the 24-hour recall, when properly done, does provide a rough estimate of a person's food consumption patterns.

3-day food diary

A better estimate of one's food intake is a *3-day food diary*. Using this method, a person writes down the food and amount eaten as it is eaten. Three days seems to be the optimum time to record one's food intake. In a shorter time period, such as one day, people tend to eat differently because they know they have to write the foods down. Longer times theoretically provide a more reliable estimate of a person's food intake; but longer records are not warranted except in research projects, because they take so much time to quantitate.

Food frequency survey

Food frequency surveys ask how often you eat an individual food or a group of foods. For instance, a typical question on a food frequency survey is, "How many times per week do you eat butter?" Food frequency surveys are used by many Wellness Centers because they are easy to administer and analyze. These surveys provide general information about the overall quality of one's diet — does one eat too many high-fat foods, too many empty calories, too few fresh fruits and vegetables? At the end of this chapter is a food frequency questionnaire that focuses on key nutrients in your diet. Complete the questionnaire to learn about your diet.

Anthropometric measurements

Anthropometric Assessments: Anthropometric measurements are measurements that can be physically determined, including *height and weight*. An individual's height is constant, but weight can very greatly with major health implications. Weight tables (most notably the Metropolitan Life Insurance Weight Tables) have been produced that give ranges of desirable weight for adult men and women. The desirable weights presented in these weight tables were determined using mortality data collected early in the 1900s. The tables were used to indicate that men or women with weight above the desirable range had an increased mortality. Most experts believe that the weights listed in these tables are too low for the current United States population since today's Americans are bigger than in 1900.

Height, weight, and frame size

The weight tables also consider a person's height and frame size. The taller a person is, the more he should weigh. Frame size (whether one has large or small bones) is also an important determinant of weight. Three frame sizes are recognized: small, medium and large. As frame size increases, the allowable weight increases. Technically, a person's frame size is determined by the width of the elbow joint when the arm is held at a 90 degree angle. An easier way to determine your frame size is to circle your wrist with the thumb and middle finger of your other hand. If the thumb and finger do not meet, then you probably have a large frame size. If the thumb and finger just meet, then you probably have a medium frame size. And if the thumb and finger overlap greatly, then you probably have a small frame size.

Body fat

More important than weight is the amount of body fat one has. There are many large people who are *overweight* (have a higher weight than is allowed for in the weight tables), such as muscular football players. There are also many people who weigh exactly what they should according to the weight tables but have an excess amount of fat. So although weight is important, the amount of body fat a person has is much more important.

Body fat is most accurately determined by very sophisticated techniques such as underwater weighing. Since it is frequently impractical to determine body fat using these techniques, alternative procedures are more commonly used. These procedures estimate percent body fat by determining *skinfold thickness* or *bioimpedence*.

Skinfold thickness determinations are one way to estimate body fat. Since much of a person's body fat is located just below the skin, measuring the skinfold thicknesses at various sites on the body allows one to calculate a person's body fat. From research using underwater weighing, formulas (such as those presented in table 2-2) were developed to estimate one's body fat by measuring various skinfold thicknesses. The more sites measured, the more accurately body fat can be determined. However, usually when measuring large numbers of people, only the triceps (back of the arm) and/or subscapular (on the back at the shoulder blade) skinfolds are measured (Figure 2-1). The skinfold thicknesses at these sites are then plugged into formulas that calculate the percent body fat. It must be emphasized that the percent body fat one determines using these formulas is only an estimate of one's actual body fat.

Figure 2-1. Sites to measure skinfold thicknesses.

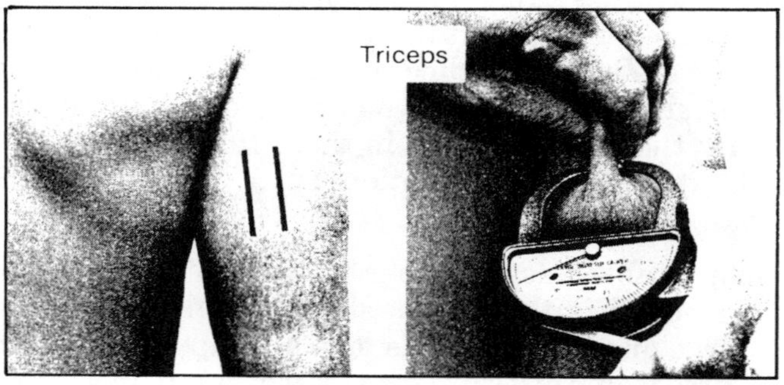

a. triceps skinfold

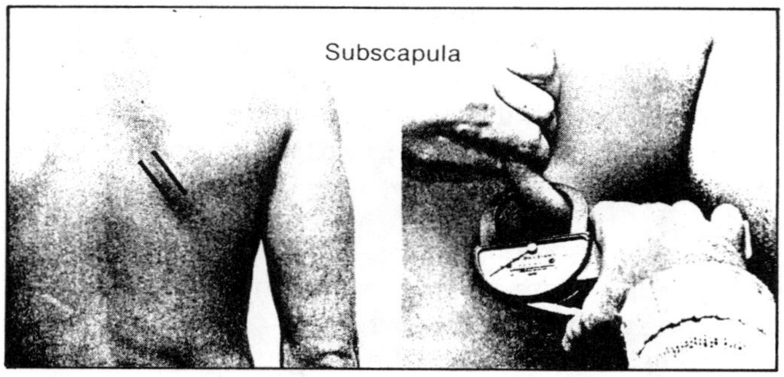

b. subscapular

From: McArdle, W.D., F.I. Katch and V.L. Katch. *Exercise Physiology: Energy, Nutrition, and Human Performance.* Lea and Febiger, Philadelphia, 1981, p. 379.

Bioimpedence is a new, high-tech method that is increasingly being used to estimate body fat. In this procedure, two electrodes are attached to a person's hand and foot. A minute electrical charge (so small that it cannot be felt) is passed through the body between these electrodes. The more fat one has, the more resistance this charge encounters in the body (fat acts like an insulator). Conversely, the more water (lean tissue — muscle and bone) in the body, the less resistance. The resistance this electrical charge encounters in the body is used (along with age, sex, height and weight) to calculate one's percent body fat. Like skinfold determinations, body fat estimates using bioimpedence should only be considered "ballpark" estimates of one's actual body fat.

Laboratory measurements

Laboratory Measurements: Whenever a nutritional assessment occurs, the nutritionist or other health professional is trained to observe the subject. The nutritionist is looking for any *physical signs* of vitamin or mineral deficiency. One cannot measure blood levels of every nutrient. However, early tell-tale warning signs of

Table 2-2. Formulas to calculate body fat in men and women.

Females:	Percent Body Fat = 0.55 × (A) + 0.31 × (B) + 6.13
Males:	Percent Body Fat = 0.43 × (A) + 0.58 × (B) + 1.47

where A = triceps skinfold (mm); B = subscapular skinfold (mm)

sub-clinical deficiencies often can be observed by noticing the subject's hair, skin, eyes and mouth. Changes in the appearance of any of these areas can be indications of underlying nutritional or other health problems.

A nutritional assessment is not complete until a number of *laboratory measurements* are made. First, blood pressure is measured. Then, generally, a sample of the subject's blood is obtained so that the following parameters can measured. Blood hemoglobin concentrations and hematocrit are determined to assess iron status. Blood cholesterol and triglyceride concentrations are determined to assess one's risk for heart disease. And blood glucose concentrations are determined to assess the occurrence of diabetes. Many other laboratory tests, including the assessment of every vitamin and mineral, can also be undertaken if thought necessary. Sometimes, especially at Wellness Centers, an exercise stress test is undertaken to determine the subject's fitness level.

From the preceding sections it is clear that a complete nutritional assessment involves many components. Some, such as blood cholesterol determinations, seemingly have little to do with nutrition. However, as people live longer, nutrition plays an increasingly large role in the occurrence of degenerative diseases. It is only after the nutritionist has all of the data from the various assessments that he is able to make nutritional recommendations.

Energy Metabolism

It is almost impossible to read a magazine or a newspaper or watch television without seeing advertisements for weight-reducing diets. Can all these claims be true? Does it really seem reasonable that you can eat all the food you want, but if you also take some pill, you will lose weight? Only by having a basic understanding of energy metabolism can one understand how ridiculous some diet claims are. This chapter will explain the components of energy expenditure. After reading this chapter, you should be able to estimate the approximate energy you expend each day. Hopefully, understanding the material in this chapter will provide information about why it is so difficult to lose weight rapidly.

Energy Intake: Every day one consumes energy in the diet. This is energy intake. Energy in the diet is expressed as *kilocalories (kcals).* While there are technical definitions of the term kilocalorie, it is simply a way to compare the energy of various foods. In the body, a pound of fat contains approximately 3500 kilocalories. Theoretically, when you eat 3500 kcals more than you expend you gain a pound of body fat. If you eat 350 kcals more than you expend every day it would take you about 10 days to gain an extra pound of fat. Or more realistically, consuming only 35 extra kcals per day translates into 3.5 pounds per year, and 35 pounds in 10 years.

Kilocalories

The macronutrients are the sources of energy in the diet. A *gram of protein* and a *gram of carbohydrate each supply 4 kilocalories* (kcal). A *gram of fat provides 9 kcals* — or over twice the energy per gram of proteins or carbohydrates. To put it another way, if one ate 100 grams (slightly less than ¼ pound) of pure protein or carbohydrate (sugar), one would consume 400 kilocalories. Eating the same weight of fat (such as butter) would provide 900 kilocalories. Except for alcohol (not considered a nutrient), which provides 7 kcals/gram, these macronutrients are the only source of energy in the diet. The vitamins and minerals, or other food components, do not provide any energy.

It is possible, if one keeps a record of the foods one eats, to calculate the energy in each food and approximate the total daily energy intake. There are food composition tables that provide an estimate of the kilocalories and other nutrients for each food. For instance, to determine the energy in a bologna sandwich one would look under "bread" to find out the kilocalories for each slice of bread. Then one would look up the energy value for a slice of bologna. Add all these values together to estimate the total energy in the sandwich. There are also computer programs available that will automatically calculate the information for each food.

Energy Expenditures: People use energy each day. This use is called energy expenditure. It is the balance between energy intake and energy expenditure that determines whether one gains or loses weight. If energy intake equals energy expenditure, a person is said to be in *energy balance* — the person is neither gaining nor losing weight. If energy intake is less than energy expenditure, then a person would lose weight; if energy intake is more than energy expenditure, the person would gain weight. All this means is that if one eats more kilocalories than one uses up in a day he will gain weight. If one wants to lose weight, then one must eat fewer kilocalories each day than he expends.

Energy balance

The energy expended by a person each day is used for one of three purposes — *basal metabolic rate, activity* and *diet-induced thermogenesis.* If one determines the amount of energy expended in each category, then the total energy expended per day can also be determined. Any determination of energy expenditures is only an approximation.

Much of the energy one uses each day maintains the *basal metabolic rate (BMR).* Energy used for basal metabolism is the minimum energy used to keep a person alive. Some of the body processes that use energy for BMR are:

BMR

1. the beating of the heart and the pumping of blood
2. body temperature regulation
3. maintenance of blood pH
4. maintenance of cellular ionic gradients
5. nerve tissue conduction
6. liver and kidney function

These are all examples of body processes that must continue if you are to stay alive. Think of them as the processes that would continue if a person were in a coma. Any activity or movement above this is not truly basal.

A person's BMR is determined in the early morning while that person is lying at rest (activity increases one's energy expenditures, even sitting up). The person should not have eaten for at least 12 hours prior to the test because the digestion, transport and storage of food increase energy expenditures (diet-induced thermogenesis). The person should be tested at a comfortable temperature and should be isolated during the test. It is only by controlling all of these factors that one can reasonably estimate basal metabolism.

Basal metabolic rate is generally determined by a method called *indirect calorimetry,* which measures a person's oxygen consumption. Since it is impossible to measure the energy directly used by a person, this substitute method was devised. The oxygen used by a person is an indication of his energy expenditures, as oxygen is used during the metabolic process. A person inspires oxygen, O_2, and expires CO_2. As the person tested breathes into a mouthpiece, the respiratory gases are collected and it is possible to determine the total volume of oxygen used over time, usually 10 minutes. Every liter of oxygen "burned" by a person is equivalent to 4.82 kilocalories.

Effect of body size on BMR

One's BMR is *directly affected by one's body size. The larger a person is, the greater the BMR.* A larger body size means more tissue to keep functioning and therefore more energy is expended in the BMR. Men, on the average, have a higher BMR than women, in part because men are bigger than women. *BMR* also *increases as lean body mass increases.* Lean body mass is a person's weight minus the weight of his adipose (fat) tissue. The more bone and muscle one has, the greater the amount of energy needed to maintain the BMR. Again, because men generally have more lean body mass than women, their BMR will be greater. It is easy to understand that a 220 pound person would have a higher BMR than a 150 pound person. However, if a man and a woman each weigh 150 pounds, the man, having a greater lean body mass than the woman, would have a higher BMR. It takes much more energy to keep muscle and bone functioning than it does to keep adipose (fat) tissue functioning.

Effect of age on BMR

A last factor that affects one's BMR is age. The *BMR decreases as one gets older.* It is estimated that a person's BMR decreases by about 10% per decade of life after age forty. That means that a person at age 75 needs only about one-half as much energy to support the BMR as when he was 25 years old. Among the reasons that BMR decreases with aging is that lean body mass also decreases with age. Even if one's weight remains the same as one gets older, there is significantly less lean body mass and more fat at the older age. Also, as you age your tissues stop functioning to the same extent as when you were younger. By age 75, your kidneys and liver are only working about 50 percent as much as when you were 25.

It would be impossible to test a large number of people using indirect calorimetry. Research on a large number of subjects has led to the development of equations using one's height, weight, age and sex, which estimate one's BMR. These equations for men and women are presented in Table 2-3. Equation 1 from Table 2-3 is a generic equation that is very easy to calculate but imprecisely estimates BMR. If the BMR of a very large population of people were determined, the average value would fit this equation. Individuals within this population might have true BMR values above or below this average. Equation 2, because it uses more data about a person to arrive at a BMR value, is more accurate than the first equation. This equation will probably provide as good an estimate of one's BMR as is possible without actually measuring the BMR.

Any movement or exercise above basal is considered energy expended in *activity*. The *energy expended in activity is proportional to a person's body weight.* The more one weighs, the more energy it takes to move this weight. It takes considerably more energy for a 200 pound person to walk a mile, than for a 100 pound person to walk the same distance. The rate at which something moves is not nearly as important as the weight which is moved. Only a small amount of extra energy is used if one runs a mile in ten minutes compared with walking a mile in twenty minutes. One can be finished running five miles a lot faster than walking five miles, but the energy expended covering this distance will not be very different. So when you think of the energy you expended in exercise, think of the weight moved and the time spent in the exercise, not the rate of movement.

Table 2-3. Equations to predict BMR in men and women.

1. BMR (kcal) = 24 × weight (kg)
2. (Men)[1] BMR (kcal) = 66.8 + 13.752(w) + 5.003(h) – 6.755(a)

   (Women)[1] BMR (kcal) = 655 + 9.563(w) + 1.850(h) – 4.67(a)

where: w = weight in kg; h = height in cm; a = age in years

1. From Linder, M.C. *Nutritional Biochemistry and Metabolism* Elsevier Science Publishing Co., New York, 1985, p. 203.

Activity and energy expenditure

Activity in one person can vary greatly on different days. The best way to estimate how much energy you spend in activity each day is to keep an activity diary. Usually activity is recorded in 10-minute segments. The energy for each activity, (i.e., walking, sitting, riding a bicycle, sleeping, etc.) is determined by taking into account your weight and the length of time each activity was undertaken. After all energy values are added, the total energy expenditure for the 24-hour period can be calculated.

An easier method that will provide a ballpark estimate of daily energy needs is presented in Table 2-4. Energy expenditure is roughly estimated based on one's category of activity. The activity categories are sedentary (not very active), moderately active, and very active. A person who is sedentary (undertakes only very light activity each day such as an office worker) could calculate his activity energy use as 30 to 40% of his BMR. The moderately active person (undertakes some regular exercise or undertakes some manual labor each day) would expend 40 to 50% of his BMR. The very active person (undertakes heavy manual labor or extensive physical exercise) might expend 50 to 100% of his BMR in daily activity. These are only gross classifications so you must use your judgment to determine your activity category. Most students' activities fall between sedentary and moderately active.

The third way energy is used is called *diet-induced thermogenesis.* This term is also referred to as the "thermic effect of food" or the "specific dynamic effect of food." What these terms mean is that it costs energy to eat foods. We eat to obtain energy for BMR and activity. However, some of the energy in the food we eat is used to *digest the food, absorb the nutrients in the food, transport the nutrients throughout the body,* and *utilize or store the nutrients.* All of these processes take energy. This means that the final energy that a food provides the body, because of diet-induced thermogenesis, is less than is actually in the food.

Thermogenesis

The energy cost of diet-induced thermogenesis is approximately 10% of the food energy one consumes. Therefore, if one eats a meal containing 1000 kcal, it costs about 100 kcal (10%) to digest, absorb, transport, and store the nutrients in that meal. The body's metabolism increases to assimilate the meal after one eats.

To calculate how much energy you spend each day in diet-induced thermogenesis, add the energy expended in BMR and activity. Since one needs to intake that much energy each day to support these processes, the energy you expend in diet-induced thermogenesis is 10% of this value.

The total energy expenditure of a person is the sum of the energy expended in BMR, activity and diet-induced thermogenesis. Table 2-4 provides examples of how this value was calculated for a 100 kg male. Table 2-4 also provides space for you to calculate your own daily energy expenditures. Even though the energy value that you obtain using this method is not exact, it will still provide you with a ballpark estimate. Most people, especially women, are amazed at how little energy they expend per day. One must consume about 3500 kilocalories less than he needs to lose one pound of fat.

If a woman having an energy expenditure of 2000 kcals (fairly average for a woman in the United States) per day reduces her energy intake to 1000 kcal per day, she will lose only about 2 pounds of fat per week. This modest weight loss is far from the weight loss of 10 to 15 pounds per week that some diet regimens advertise. Even if the woman stops eating altogether, at most she will only lose about 4 pounds of fat per week. However, as discussed in the next chapter, if one consumes too few calories per day, the body adjusts by reducing its energy expended in the BMR. Thus, it is very difficult by dieting alone to lose weight rapidly. One should attempt to lose weight very slowly by reducing caloric intake only slightly (less than 500 kcals per day) and increasing one's exercise. Remember that one gains weight slowly and this is how one should attempt to lose it.

In conclusion, before nutritional recommendations can be made, a complete nutritional assessment should be undertaken. This includes medical and family histories, anthropometric assessment, dietary analysis, and laboratory measurements. It is only after a complete assessment is conducted that one can make valid nutritional suggestions. A determination of one's daily energy consumption will often reveal that one is not as active as he might believe. When one does not expend very many calories daily, it is difficult by dieting alone to lose weight rapidly. This chapter provided ways to estimate your energy expenditures.

Table 2-4. Calculation of daily total energy expenditure.

EXAMPLE: 220 pound male; 6 ft 3 in tall; 24 years old; mod. active

1. Calculate BMR

   BMR = 24 × 100 (kg) = 2400 kcal/day

2. Calculate Activity (moderately active)

   Activity = 45% of BMR = 0.45 × 2400 kcal/day = 1080 kcal/day

3. Calculate Diet-induced Thermogenesis

   1. Add energy from BMR and Activity together
   2. Multiply by 10%

   Thermogenesis = 2400 + 1080 = 3580 × 0.10 = 358 kcal/day

Total Energy Expenditure = BMR + Activity + Thermogenesis = 2400 + 1080 + 358 = 3838 kcal/day

---

Calculate your daily energy expenditure:

A. weight _____ lbs (divide by 2.2 to change to kg)= _____ kg

B. height _____ inches (multiply by 2.54 to change to cm) _____ cm

C. age _____ years

D. activity: light (30-40% of BMR)

   moderately active (40-50% of BMR)

   very active (50-100% of BMR)

1. BMR = 24 × _____ weight (kg) = _____ kcal
2. Activity = BMR _____ × _____% = _____ kcal
3. Thermogenesis = BMR _____ + Activity _____ × 0.10 = _____ kcal

Total Energy Expenditures = BMR + Activity + Thermogenesis =

_____ + _____ + _____ = _____ kcal/day

ILLUSTRATION: LOEL BARR

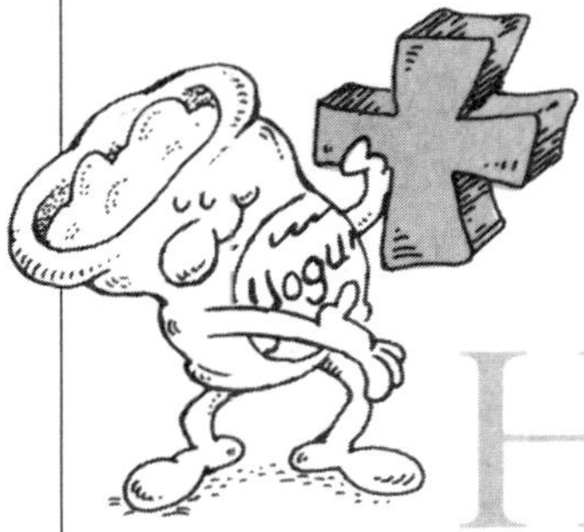

How's Your Diet?

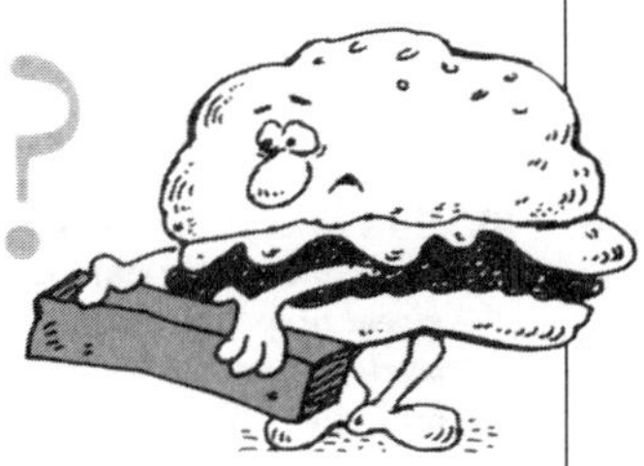

The 42 questions below will help you focus on the key features of your diet. The (+) or (−) numbers under each set of answers instantly pat you on the back for good habits or alert you to problems you may not even realize you have. (Sorry.)

The Grand Total rates your overall diet, on a scale from "Super" to "Arghh!"

The quiz focuses on fat, sodium, sugar, fiber, and vitamins A and C. It doesn't attempt to cover everything in your diet. Also, it doesn't attempt to measure precisely *how much* of these key nutrients you eat.

What the quiz *will* do is give you a rough sketch of your current eating habits and, implicitly, suggest what you can do to improve them.

Finally, please don't despair over a less-than-perfect score. A healthy diet isn't built overnight.

INSTRUCTIONS

- Under each answer is a number with a + or − sign in front of it. Circle the number that is directly beneath the answer you choose. That's your score for the question. (If you use a pencil, you can erase your answers and give the quiz to a friend or relative.)
- Circle only one number for each question, unless the instructions tell you to "average two or more scores if necessary."
- How to average. In answering question 19, for example, if you drink fruit juice (+1) and coffee (−1) on a typical day, add the two scores (which gives you 0) and then divide by 2. That gives you a score of 0 for the question. If averaging gives you a fraction, round it off to the nearest whole number.
- Make sure you pay attention to serving sizes. For example, a serving of vegetables is ½ cup. If you usually eat one cup of vegetables at a time, count it as two servings.
- Add up all your + scores, and write the total in the *Total (+)* column at the end of the quiz.
- Add up all your − scores, and write the total in the *Total (−)* column at the end of the quiz.
- Subtract the *Total (−)* column from the *Total (+)* column. That will give you your GRAND TOTAL.

QUIZ

1. How many times per week do you eat unprocessed red meat (steak, roast beef, lamb or pork chops, burgers, etc.)?

(a) 1 or less +3 (b) 2-3 +2 (c) 4-5 −1 (d) 6 or more −3

2. After cooking, how large is the serving of red meat you usually eat? *(To convert from raw to cooked, reduce by 25 percent. For example, 4 oz. of raw meat shrinks to 3 oz. after cooking. There are 16 oz. in a pound.)*

(a) 8 oz. or more −3 (b) 6-7 oz. −1 (c) 4-5 oz. +1

(d) 3 oz. or less +3 (e) don't eat +3

3. Do you trim the visible fat when you cook or eat red meat?

(a) yes +3 (b) no −3 (c) don't eat red meat +3

4. How many times per week do you eat processed meats (hot dogs, bacon, sausage, bologna, luncheon meats, etc.)?

(a) none +3 (b) less than 1 +2 (c) 1-2 0 (d) 3-4 −1 (e) 5 or more −3

5. What kind of ground meat or poultry do you usually eat?

(a) regular ground beef −3 (b) lean ground beef −2

(c) extra-lean ground beef −1 (d) ground round 0

(e) ground turkey +1 (f) don't eat +3

6. What type of bread do you usually eat?

(a) whole wheat or other whole grain +3 (b) rye +2

(c) pumpernickel +2 (d) white, "wheat," French, or Italian −2

7. How many times per week do you eat deep-fried foods (fish, chicken, vegetables, potatoes, etc.)?

(a) none +3 (b) 1-2 0 (c) 3-4 −1 (d) 5 or more −3

8. How many servings of vegetables do you eat per day? *(One serving = ½ cup. Include non-fried potatoes.)*

(a) none −3 (b) 1 0 (c) 2 +1 (d) 3 +2 (e) 4 or more +3

9. How many servings of cruciferous vegetables do you usually eat per week? *(ONLY count kale, broccoli, cauliflower, cabbage, Brussels sprouts, greens, bok choy, kohlrabi, turnip, and rutabaga. One serving = ½ cup.)*

(a) none −3 (b) 1-3 +1 (c) 4-6 +2 (d) 7 or more +3

ILLUSTRATION: LOEL BARR

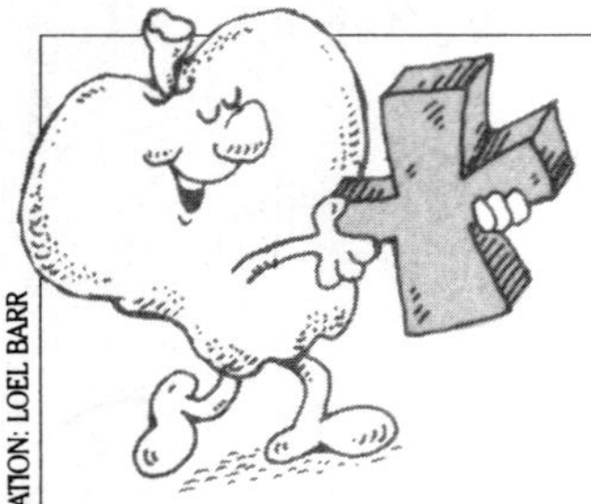

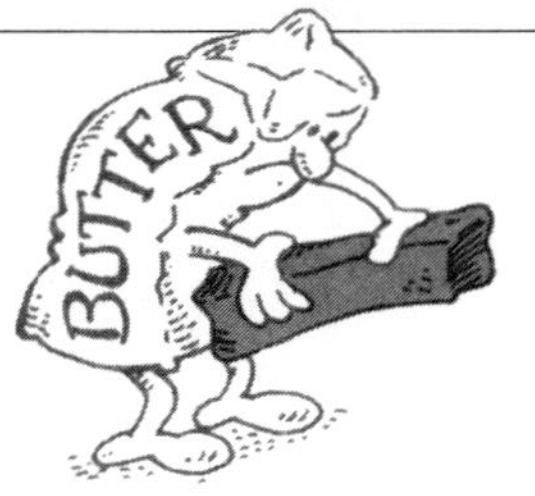

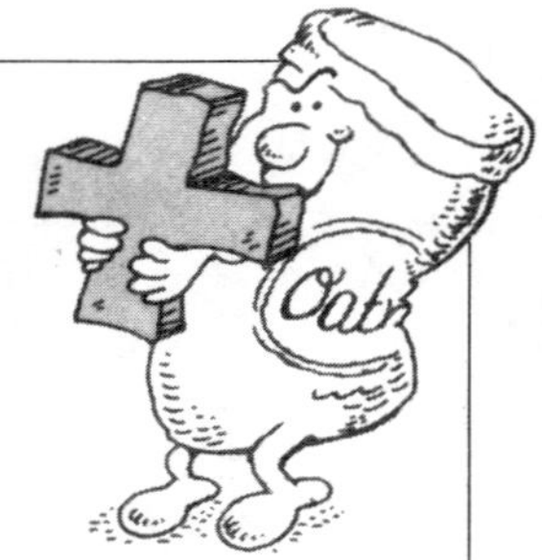

10. How many servings of vitamin-A-rich fruits or vegetables do you usually eat per week? ***(ONLY count carrots, pumpkin, sweet potatoes, cantaloupe, spinach, winter squash, greens, apricots, and broccoli. One serving = ½ cup.)***
(a) none −3 (b) 1-3 +1 (c) 4-6 +2 (d) 7 or more +3

11. How many times per week do you eat at a fast-food restaurant? ***(Include burgers, fried fish or chicken, croissant or biscuit sandwiches, topped potatoes, and other main dishes. Omit meals of just plain baked potato, broiled chicken, or salad.)***
(a) none +3 (b) less than 1 +1 (c) 1 0 (d) 2 −1 (e) 3 −2 (f) 4 or more −3

12. How many servings of grains rich in complex carbohydrates do you eat per day? ***(One serving = 1 slice of bread, 1 large pancake, or ½ cup cooked cereal, rice, pasta, bulgur, wheat berries, kasha, or millet. Omit heavily-sweetened cold cereals.)***
(a) none −3 (b) 1-2 0 (c) 3-4 +1 (d) 5-6 +2 (e) 7 or more +3

13. How many servings of beer, wine, or liquor do you drink? ***(Count as one serving: 12 oz. regular or light beer, 4 oz. wine, or 1 oz. liquor.)***
(a) 1 or less a week +3 (b) 2-3 a week +1 (c) 4-7 a week 0
(d) 2 a day −2 (e) more than 2 a day −3

14. How many times per week do you eat fish or shellfish? ***(Omit deep-fried items, tuna packed in oil, shrimp, squid, and mayonnaise-laden tuna salad—a little mayo is okay.)***
(a) none −2 (b) 1-2 +1 (c) 3-4 +2 (d) 5 or more +3

15. How many times per week do you eat cheese? ***(Include pizza, cheeseburgers, veal or eggplant parmigiana, cream cheese, etc. Omit lowfat or "lite" cheeses.)***
(a) 1 or less +3 (b) 2-3 +2 (c) 4-5 −1 (d) 6 or more −3

16. How many servings of fresh fruit do you consume per day?
(a) none −3 (b) 1 0 (c) 2 +1 (d) 3 +2 (e) 4 or more +3

17. Do you remove the skin before eating poultry?
(a) yes +3 (b) no −3 (c) don't eat poultry +3

18. What do you usually put on your bread or toast? ***(Average two or more scores if necessary.)***
(a) butter −3 (b) cream cheese −3 (c) margarine −2 (d) diet margarine −1
(e) jam 0 (f) fruit butter +3 (g) nothing +3

19. Which of these beverages do you drink on a typical day? ***(Average two or more scores if necessary.)***
(a) fruit juice +1 (b) water or club soda +3 (c) diet soda −1
(d) coffee or tea −1 (e) soda or fruit drink or ade −3

20. How many servings of caffeine-containing beverages do you drink per day? ***(One serving = 1 cup of coffee or tea, or 12 oz. of cola.)***
(a) none +3 (b) 1 +1 (c) 2 −1 (d) 3 −2 (e) 4 or more −3

21. Which flavorings do you most frequently add to your foods? ***(Average two or more scores if necessary.)***
(a) garlic or lemon juice +3 (b) herbs or spices +3 (c) soy sauce −2
(d) margarine −2 (e) salt −3 (f) butter −3 (g) nothing +3

22. What do you eat most frequently as a snack? ***(Average two or more scores if necessary.)***
(a) fruits or vegetables +3 (b) sweetened yogurt +2 (c) nuts −1
(d) chips −2 (e) cookies −2 (f) granola bar −2 (g) candy bar −3
(h) pastry −3 (i) nothing 0

23. What is your most typical breakfast? ***(Subtract an extra 3 points if you also eat bacon or sausage.)***
(a) croissant, danish, or doughnut −3 (b) eggs −3 (c) pancakes or waffles −2
(d) nothing 0 (e) cereal or bread +3 (f) yogurt or cottage cheese +3

24. What do you usually eat for dessert?
(a) pie, pastry, or cake −3 (b) ice cream −3 (c) yogurt, ice milk, or sorbet +1
(d) fruit +3 (e) nothing +3

25. How many times per week do you eat beans, split peas, or lentils?
(a) none −2 (b) 1 +1 (c) 2 +2 (d) 3 or more +3

26. What kind of milk do you drink?
(a) whole −3 (b) 2% lowfat −1 (c) 1% lowfat +2 (d) ½% or skim +3 (e) none 0

27. What dressings or toppings do you usually add to your salads? ***(ADD two or more scores if necessary.)***
(a) nothing, lemon, or vinegar +3 (b) reduced-calorie dressing +1
(c) regular dressing −1 (d) croutons or bacon bits −1
(e) cole slaw, pasta salad, or potato salad −1

28. What sandwich fillings do you eat most frequently? ***(Average two or more scores if necessary.)***
(a) luncheon meat −3 (b) cheese or roast beef −1 (c) peanut butter 0
(d) tuna, salmon, chicken, or turkey +3

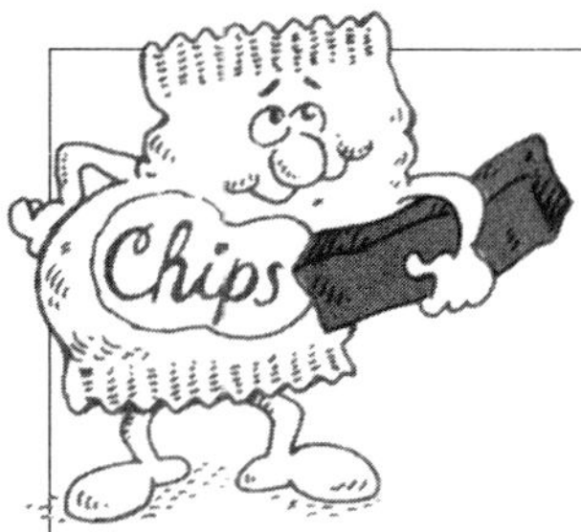

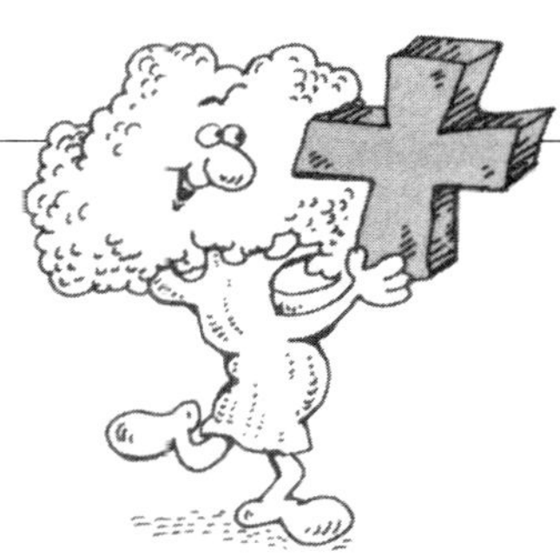

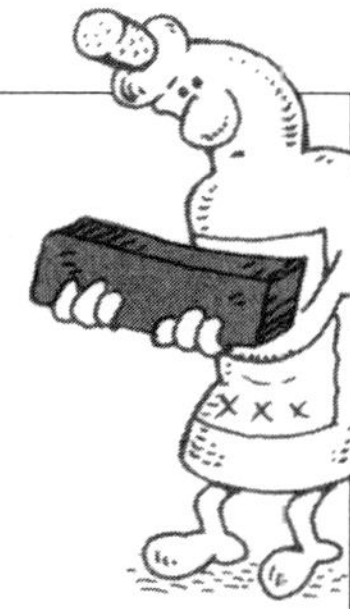

ILLUSTRATION: LOEL BARR

29. What do you usually spread on your sandwiches? ***(Average two or more scores if necessary.)***
(a) mayonnaise −2 (b) light mayonnaise −1 (c) mustard 0
(d) ketchup 0 (e) nothing +3

30. How many egg yolks do you eat per week? ***(Add 1 yolk for every slice of quiche you eat.)***
(a) 2 or less +3 (b) 3-4 +2 (c) 5-6 +1 (d) 7 or more −3

31. How many times per week do you eat canned or dried soups? ***(Omit low-sodium, lowfat soups.)***
(a) none +3 (b) 1-2 0 (c) 3-4 −2 (d) 5 or more −3

32. How many servings of a rich source of calcium do you eat per day? ***(One serving = ⅔ cup milk or yogurt, 1 oz. cheese, 1½ oz. sardines, 3½ oz. salmon, 5 oz. tofu, 1 cup greens or broccoli, or 200 mg of a calcium supplement.)***
(a) none −3 (b) 1 +1 (c) 2 +2 (d) 3 or more +3

33. What do you usually order on your pizza? ***(Non-meat toppings include green pepper, mushrooms, onions, and other vegetables. Subtract 1 extra point if you order extra cheese.)***
(a) no cheese w/non-meat toppings +3
(b) cheese w/non-meat toppings +1 (c) cheese 0
(d) cheese w/meat toppings −3 (e) don't eat pizza +2

34. What kind of cookies do you usually eat?
(a) graham crackers +1 (b) ginger snaps +1 (c) oatmeal −1
(d) chocolate coated, chocolate chip, or peanut butter −3
(e) sandwich cookies (like Oreos) −3 (f) don't eat cookies +3

35. What kind of frozen dessert do you usually eat? ***(Subtract 1 extra point for each topping—whipped cream, hot fudge, nuts, etc.)***
(a) gourmet ice cream −3 (b) regular ice cream −1
(c) sorbet, sherbet, or ices +1 (d) frozen yogurt or ice milk +1
(e) don't eat frozen desserts +3

36. What kind of cake or pastry do you usually eat?
(a) cheesecake, pie, or any microwave cake −3
(b) cake with frosting or filling −2
(c) cake without frosting −1 (d) angelfood cake +1
(e) unfrosted muffin, banana bread, or carrot cake 0
(f) don't eat cakes or pastries +3

37. How many times per week does your dinner contain grains, vegetables, or beans, but little or no animal protein (meat, poultry, fish, eggs, milk, or cheese)?
(a) none −1 (b) 1 +1 (c) 2 +2 (d) 3 +3

38. Which of the following salty snacks do you typically eat?
(a) potato chips or packaged popcorn −3 (b) tortilla chips −1
(c) light potato chips −2 (d) salted pretzels −1 (e) unsalted pretzels +1
(f) homemade air-popped popcorn +3 (g) don't eat +3

39. What do you usually use to sauté vegetables or other foods? ***(Vegetable oil includes safflower, corn, canola, olive, sunflower, and soybean.)***
(a) butter or lard −3
(b) more than one tablespoon of margarine or vegetable oil −1
(c) no more than one tablespoon of margarine or vegetable oil +1
(d) water or broth +3

40. What kind of cereal do you usually eat?
(a) hot whole-grain (like oatmeal or Wheatena) +3
(b) cold whole-grain (like Shredded Wheat) +3
(c) cold low-fiber (like Corn Flakes) 0
(d) sugary cold low-fiber (like Frosted Flakes) −1 (e) granola −2

41. With what do you make tuna salad, pasta salad, chicken salad, etc?
(a) mayonnaise −2 (b) light mayonnaise 0
(c) lowfat yogurt +2 (d) nonfat yogurt +3

42. What do you typically put on your pasta? ***(Add one point if you also add sauteed vegetables. Average two or more scores if necessary.)***
(a) tomato-based sauce +3 (b) tomato sauce with a little parmesan +3
(c) white clam sauce +1 (d) meat sauce −1
(e) tomato sauce with meatballs −2 (f) Alfredo, or other creamy sauce −3

Total (+) ________ **Total (−)** ________

YOUR GRAND TOTAL ________

+73 to +127	SUPER!	You're a nutrition superstar. Give yourself a big (non-butter) pat on the back.
+30 to +72	GOOD	Pin your Quiz to a wall or bulletin board (with your name in large print, of course.)
−14 to +29	FAIR	Hang in there. Tape CSPI's Nutrition Scoreboard poster to your refrigerator for a little friendly help.
−123 to −15	ARGHH!	Stop lining the cat box with *Nutrition Action Healthletter.* Empty your refrigerator and cupboard. It's time to start over.

Name ____________________

Section ____________________

Date ____________________

Chapter 2
QUESTIONS FOR REVIEW

1. List three forms of diet histories used in nutritional assessment.

   a. 24 hr recall

   b. food diary (3 days)

   c. food frequency

2. Anthropometric measurements are measurements that can be physically determined. They include wt and ht.

3. List the factors used to determine a person's ideal body weight.

   a. sex

   b. wt

   c. body frame

   d.

4. A person could be overweight but not overfat (TRUE? FALSE?)

5. What are two methods used to estimate body fat?

   a. Skinfold method

   b. bioimpedence

6. List three laboratory measurements that are used to assess a person's health status.

   a.

   b.

   c.

7. Dietary energy is expressed in ____________________ .

8. In the body, a pound of fat contains approximately __________ kilocalories.

9. How many kilocalories do each of the macronutrients supply (per gram)?

   a. protein ______________ kcals/gram

   b. carbohydrate ______________ kcals/gram

   c. fat ______________ kcals/gram

   d. alcohol (not a nutrient) ______________ kcals/gram

10. List the three ways the body expends energy each day.

    a.

    b.

    c.

11. The basal metabolic rate (BMR) is higher/lower in a large person than in a small person. The BMR increases/decreases as one gets older. The more muscle one has the higher/lower the BMR.

12. The energy used in activity increases/decreases as one's size increases.

13. Dietary-induced thermogenesis accounts for about 10/20/30 percent of one's energy expended each day.

CHAPTER 3

Overweight and Underweight

National surveys show that very few people in the United States are satisfied with their body weight. Although some people think they are too thin, in today's world most people, rightly or wrongly, believe that they are overweight. Unfortunately, for those who would like to lose weight there is no easy way to do it. And therein lies the problem. Most people gain weight slowly over a period of years. However, they try to lose it rapidly. One recent publication estimated that over 29,000 different diet schemes have been introduced in the last thirty years. Does it seem likely that if any of these plans or pills were successful there would be any need to introduce any new plans? This chapter discusses the occurrence and health ramifications of obesity. The components that must be integrated into any diet to lose weight are also discussed. Finally, the increasing occurrence of the eating disorders anorexia nervosa and bulimia in our society today are discussed.

It is estimated that there are over 29,000 diet plans available.

Obesity: Obesity can be defined in different ways. Regardless of how it is defined, it is an excess accumulation of adipose tissue (fat). Stricter definitions use a person's ideal body weight from height/weight tables (discussed in Chapter 2) to categorize people. Using these criteria, *overweight is defined as 110 to 120 percent of ideal body weight (IBW). Obesity is defined as greater than 120 percent of IBW.* Many nutritionists believe that these values are too low for several reasons. First, Americans are bigger today than ever before. Also, many muscular people exceed 120 percent of IBW but would hardly be considered obese. And finally, some people may be at their desired weight but may be excessively fat. It is therefore very difficult to categorize a person on the basis of weight alone.

Obesity is an excess accumulation of adipose tissue (fat).

Obesity is a concern in today's society because it is related to many health problems. As weight increases, so does the occurrence of *diabetes, gout, gallbladder disease, hypertension, joint disease and arthritis,* and *blood cholesterol (increased risk of heart disease).* While not all of these problems are present in every obese person, it is clear that the more one weighs the more likely one is to experience one or more of these problems. How overweight does one have to be before the above-mentioned problems develop? It varies among individuals. In some people only a slight increase in weight leads to health problems while others seem not to be affected by moderate excess weight. Unless a specific health problem exists, many physicians do not become too concerned about body weight until one exceeds 140 to 150 percent of IBW. It also appears that if an obese person can remain very active the occurrence of health problems is greatly lessened. To remain active as one gains weight is not easy, because as people gain weight they tend to become more inactive, which in turn causes them to gain more weight, leading to a vicious cycle. Thus, activity or the lack of it, as much as obesity, sometimes contributes to the medical problems of the obese.

Gross obesity is defined as 200% of IBW

One category of obesity which undeniably causes ill health is gross obesity. Gross obesity is defined as obesity in excess of 200 percent of IBW. People that weigh more than twice their normal body weight have a much-increased occurrence of the medical problems previously discussed. In addition, the grossly obese often suffer from shortness of breath (because they have difficulty in moving their chest muscles to breathe) and sleep apnea (the tendency to fall asleep at any time). Gross obesity also relates to an inability to breathe properly. The grossly obese often cannot sleep lying down because the weight of the chest makes it impossible to breathe.

Dieting and Weight Loss: There are many reasons for obesity. It is possible to document cultural, behavioral and metabolic reasons for obesity. Since obesity has many causes, it is naive to think that any single gimmick diet can actually cure obesity. Any diet plan that says that dieting is easy, rapid, or that a person can eat all foods and still lose weight just is not realistic. It is possible to lose weight rapidly, by consuming very low-calorie diets. However, that weight loss is mostly water and/or protein — not fat. The goal of dieting is to lose body fat, not muscle. This can only be done over a slow period by moderately reducing one's dietary calories.

Another point to consider is that the goal of dieting is not only to lose weight but to keep the weight off. It is relatively easier to lose weight using some of the fad diets than it is to keep the weight off. Generally, the faster a person tries to lose weight, the faster the weight returns; sometimes the person gains even more than he began with. Any diet undertaken must not only consider weight loss, but also lifelong maintenance of weight after the loss.

Most research shows that less than 25 percent of people dieting actually lose more than 25 pounds of weight. And less than 15 percent keep the weight off for more than one year. Table 3-1 provides information about the components of every reasonable diet plan.

Consumption of less than 1200 kcals/day is dangerous.

It is necessary to reduce calories in order to lose weight. However, one should never consume less than 1200 kcals per day. Diets containing less than 1200 kcals per day are dangerous. They cause excessive protein loss from the body (including the heart) and other dangerous metabolic changes. Very low-calorie diet regimens such as "Optifast" must only be undertaken with a physician's supervision. The use of these low-calorie diets is only justified in people who are very obese.

For the best long-term results, one should only *reduce dietary calories to about 500 less than needed each day.* When one makes large reductions in his caloric intake, the body adjusts by decreasing the energy used in basal metabolism (BMR). When you decrease your dietary calories too much, the body, as a survival mechanism, decreases your energy expenditures. When you reduce your calories it is very important that you *eat foods from a variety of sources.* Do not limit your diet to just a few foods. You cannot get all of the nutrients that you need that way.

Table 3-1. Necessary components of a diet plan.

1. Modest reduction in dietary calories
2. Increase in energy expended in exercise
3. Behavior modification to change eating habits to maintain desirable weight

Exercise is also a necessary part of any plan to lose weight. Exercise increases one's energy expenditure. Depending on body weight (the more you weigh, the more you expend), one expends up to 500 kcals by walking three miles per day. Thus, expending an extra 500 kcals per day in exercise can double the energy deficit per day if one also decreases his dietary calories by 500 kilocalories. Exercise also causes protein to be retained in the body, or to be lost more slowly. Exercise slows down the body's tendency to decrease its BMR when less calories than are needed are consumed. Exercise, therefore, should be an integral part of any weight-reducing plan.

You cannot properly lose weight without exercise.

The last component of any weight-reduction regimen should be *behavior modification.* Often people go to weight-reducing spas. Many of these programs are very successful at helping people lose weight. The best of these programs integrate nutritional counseling with exercise and behavior modification. However, in most of the cases, after the person leaves he returns to the same environment with the same stresses and lifestyle that contributed to his obesity initially. The prognosis in such cases is not promising. To be really successful, not just at losing weight but at keeping the weight off, one must change his eating habits. In most cases, this means to substitute fresh fruits and vegetables for snack foods. It also means eliminating between-meals snacks, especially evening snacks. Food diaries should be kept. The person should not only write down the foods that he consumes each time he eats, but also any stress that contributed to the eating of the foods. If a person is unsuccessful at changing his food consumption patterns after dieting, he will most likely be unsuccessful maintaining his new weight.

Yo-Yo Dieting Syndrome: Recent research has shown that repetitive dieting can cause a person to gain weight. That's right —the more a person diets, the more he ends up weighing! This phenomenon has been called "Yo-Yo dieting syndrome."

To understand why dieting causes one to gain weight it is necessary to look at the components of weight loss during dieting. The progression of weight changes during dieting is shown in Table 3-2.

Yo-Yo dieting can actually result in weight gain.

Table 3-2. Stages of weight changes during dieting.

Stage 1	Initial, rapid weight loss phase
Stage 2	Steady weight loss phase
Stage 3	Plateau phase
Stage 4	Regain phase

As has been conclusively shown in animal experiments, when a person cuts his caloric consumption the body reduces its energy needed for the BMR. After about a month or so of dieting, one's weight loss slows down. This is called the "plateau phase" of weight loss. This plateau phase occurs even though the dieter consumes the same number of calories that caused rapid weight-loss during the early part of dieting. By this time most people stop dieting (they get discouraged, etc.). Upon going back to their regular food-consumption patterns (higher caloric intake), most people regain the weight faster than they lost it. This weight gain occurs because the body does not (or cannot) increase the BMR when one returns to his normal diet. After dieting, a person is much more metabolically efficient than before dieting — less food is perceived by the body as more food.

Each time a person goes through one of these cycles he appears to become more metabolically efficient. (Figure 3-1). Each time a person re-diets it takes longer and longer to lose the same amount of weight. And that person regains the weight more quickly, usually ending up at a greater weight than he began with. The only way to prevent this from happening is to maintain one's new, lower body weight for some period of time (at least three years) after the diet.

Figure 3-1. Yo-Yo Diet Syndrome

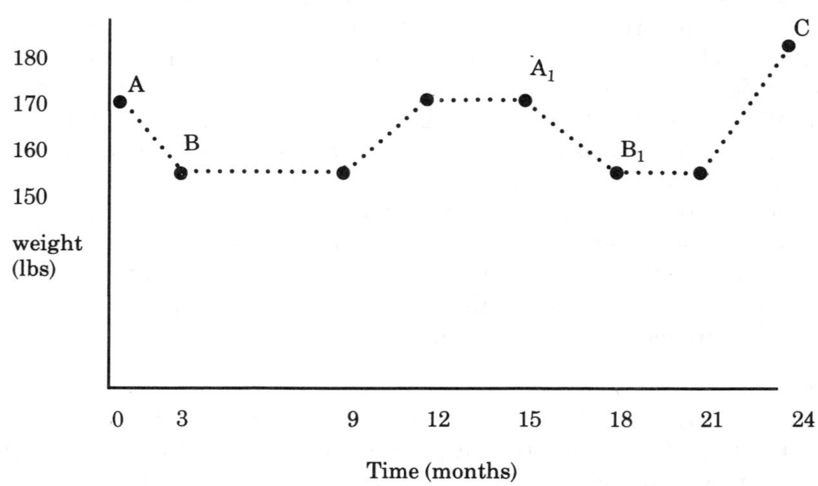

A Woman weighing 170 pounds starts 1000 kcal/day diet
B Ends diet (usually due to very slow weight loss)
A_1 Restarts 1000 kcal/day diet
B_1 Ends diet (weight loss slower than first diet)
C Regains lost weight and more. Final weight 180+ pounds.

An easy-to-understand plan to slowly lose weight is called the "rule of 10." The concept is that to lose weight slowly one must only moderately reduce his calories. To determine the minimum kilocalories that a person should consume each day, a woman should multiply her weight (in pounds) by 10. A man, being a little larger, should multiply his weight by 12. Thus, a woman weighing 180 pounds should eat at least 1800 kilocalories (10 times 180 pounds) per day. In addition to this moderate caloric decrease per day, one following this plan should also try to exercise for 20-30 minutes extra per day. This very modest decrease in food energy consumed, and modest increase in energy expended per day will result in slow, but steady, weight loss — as much as 25 pounds per year. Remember, you only gain weight slowly, and to try to lose it too fast is not effective in the long run.

The Rule of 10

To reiterate, weight loss should be slow with modest decreases in one's daily caloric consumption. Exercise should be an integral part of one's weight-reducing regimen, as exercise contributes to the caloric deficit and helps prevent the BMR from being shut down. Weight reduction is only the first step; one needs to keep the weight off. This can be accomplished best by lifestyle changes that affect exercise and food consumption patterns. If you lose weight too rapidly the body tends to want to regain that weight by becoming more efficient. Thus, to avoid the "Yo-Yo syndrome," diet slowly, increase your exercise, and change your food habits.

Anorexia Nervosa: Anorexia nervosa is an eating disorder whose incidence is increasing in the United States. Twenty years ago, it was thought that about one female in 800-1000 might be afflicted with the disease. It is now estimated that one female in 400-500 has the disease. Twenty years ago three of every four persons diagnosed died from anorexia. While we have made much progress, approximately one in every four persons diagnosed with anorexia dies. It is important to recognize the symptoms of anorexia because a person afflicted with this disease must seek professional help.

Estimates are that 1 out of every 400-500 females has Anorexia Nervosa.

Anorexia nervosa afflicts primarily young females from affluent families. In fact, the disease only occurs in the affluent nations of the world. The typical young woman is from a family in which the father is very successful and very demanding.

There are several criteria for establishing anorexia. First, if a person loses more than 25 percent of her body weight, anorexia is strongly indicated. Also, any person whose body weight is less than 80 percent of ideal body weight should also be suspected of anorexia. Family physicians chart body weight and stature (height) during office visits until a person is 18 years of age. Deviations in weight from a person's norm without corresponding deviations in height are indicative of developing anorexia.

Physicians are much more aware of this problem today than they have been in the past. If a problem is suspected, very sophisticated measurement can conclusively diagnose anorexia nervosa.

There are other symptoms besides weight loss that suggest a person may be anorexic. First, the anorexic has a *distorted attitude about foods.* She does not differentiate between the caloric-content of

To the anorexic, all foods are bad, even good ones.

high-calorie and low-calorie foods. To the anorexic, all foods are bad and cause weight-gain. Second, the anorexic *denies her illness*. She does not, even while starving to death, believe that there is anything wrong with her. Third, the anorexic has a *distorted body image.* No matter how thin the anorexic becomes, she does not think she is thin enough.

Eventually, as the anorexic loses weight, the reduced body weight produces clinical symptóms. These symptoms include *lanugo* (downy hair growth over the body), *amenorrhea* (cessation of the menstrual cycle), *postural hypotension* (dizziness, or fainting upon standing), *tachycardia* (rapid heartbeat), and *edema* (water accumulation in the arms and the legs). Once edema starts to occur the anorexic is very seriously ill, and under most circumstances must be hospitalized.

Treatment of anorexia nervosa takes the form of psychological counseling. Anorexia nervosa is not really a nutritional problem; it is a psychological problem that has a food component. The first step in treating the anorexic is *nutritional supplementation.* Frequently this requires hospitalization. Most often the person must be fed parenterally (tube-fed). The patient must be carefully watched so that she does not remove the tubes from her arm. After she has been nutritionally stabilized, long-term *behavior therapy* must be undertaken. The person must develop a different attitude about herself. Lastly, *group family therapy* is recommended. The person must come to understand her role in the family unit, what is expected of her, and what support she can expect from her family. Anorexia nervosa is most successfully treated when it is diagnosed early. The prognosis is much bleaker if the disease progresses to the stage at which the patient must be hospitalized.

Bulimia — binge eating

Bulimia: Bulimia, also called the binge/purge syndrome, is another disease of affluence. Everyone binges (eats more food than they want to) occasionally. True bulimia only occurs when excessive intake becomes recurrent or addictive. Bulimmia occurs more frequently in women than in men (the ratio is about 5 women to every 1 man). Studies have estimated that on some college campuses as many as 20 percent of the women and 5 percent of the men students have undergone at least one binge/purge episode. The estimate of those that could be considered true addictive bulimics is much lower — 5 and 1 percent of the women and men, respectively — but still alarming.

One cannot recognize a bulimic by body size or shape. *A bulimic can be thin, normal weight or obese*. Recent studies have shown, however, that most bulimics are somewhat overweight. Other characteristics of the bulimic are that they *feel guilty when binging*, they are *secretive*, and they are *aware of their abnormal eating pattern, but can do nothing about it*, and they often *undergo large weight fluctuations*. The bulimic consumes high-calorie, high-sugar and high-fat foods during a binge. As many as 15,000 calories can be consumed during a binge (15,000 calories would be equivalent to eating more than 20 Big Macs).

Bulimia is addictive. Mood changes occur during binging. Often the bulimic ends the binge because she goes to sleep. Binging tends to be calming, causing the release of brain neurochemicals. When a person becomes anxious, he binges to calm down — even though he knows this is not normal. Thus, the process becomes addictive.

Because the bulimic knows that the consumption of tremendously large amounts of calories is dangerous, he often purges to rid himself of these calories. Purging takes one of two forms. The most common form of purging is self-induced vomiting. Another form of purging is excessive laxative use. Both of these types of purging are very dangerous, especially if continued for a long period of time. The medical problems associated with bulimia are listed in Table 3-3.

Purging with excess vomiting or over-use of laxatives is common but extremely dangerous.

The medical problems of bulimia are very real, and sometimes life-threatening. If the esophagus or stomach ruptures it is usually fatal. Because of fluid losses during vomiting, a great many minerals (especially potassium) are lost from the body. If the body is depleted of too much potassium or any other mineral, major medical problems such as the inability to maintain blood pH, or heart arrythmias, can occur. In fact, the heart could stop if the imbalances become severe enough. Excessive loss of dental enamel from stomach acid can significantly accelerate the course of tooth decay. Dentists are now aware of this fact and watch for it in their patients.

Excessive laxative use can also be very dangerous. First, laxatives do not significantly decrease the digestion and absorption of nutrients from the diet. Often bulimics are operating under a misconception when they think that laxatives will decrease the body's assimilation of nutrients. Second, if used all the time, one needs to consume larger and larger doses of laxative for them to remain effective. Laxatives also cause large amounts of minerals to be lost from the body, especially potassium. Again, these mineral imbalances are very serious. Lastly, excessive use of laxatives causes the colon to stop working (cathartic colon) except in the presence of more laxative.

Table 3-3. Major medical problems associated with bulimia.

1. Medical problems associated with binging
   a. obesity — from excess calories
   b. gastric rupturing — stomach bursts from too much food
2. Medical problems associated with vomiting
   a. heartburn — from reflux of stomach acid into esophagus
   b. esophageal rupture
   c. tooth decay — acid from stomach destroys teeth enamel
   d. metabolic alkalosis
   e. heart arrythmias
3. Medical problems associated with excessive laxative use
   a. dehydration
   b. constipation
   c. mineral imbalances — excess loss of potassium in feces
   d. cathartic colon — colon needs more and more laxative to work

Psychoanalysis is the treatment for bulimia.

The treatment of the bulimic is, like that of the anorexic, rooted in psychoanalysis. The bulimic must undergo behavior therapy and individual psychological counseling to overcome this problem. Unlike the anorexic, the outlook is fairly promising.

Because the problems of anorexia nervosa and bulimia occur much more frequently on college campuses, most colleges have counselors that have been trained to deal with these problems. If you have a problem, seek a counselor (usually at the campus infirmary). Or if you suspect someone suffers from either of these problems, urge him or her to seek help. Neither of these problems will go away.

Calories Don't Count...Equally

BY BONNIE LIEBMAN

A calorie is a calorie. So goes the adage. But a growing body of evidence suggests that once a calorie enters the body, this simple rule of dieting dogma isn't always true.

Instead, fat calories may be particularly good at making fat bodies. And people who have lost weight may be especially "hungry" for the fatty foods that will do their diets in. What's worse, their bodies may be primed to store every bite of incoming fat, rather than burn it for energy.

Why some people gain weight and others stay slim is still a puzzle. It has no easy, and probably no single, solution. Yet many researchers now agree that if any diet is going to help take *and keep* weight off, it's got to be low in fat.

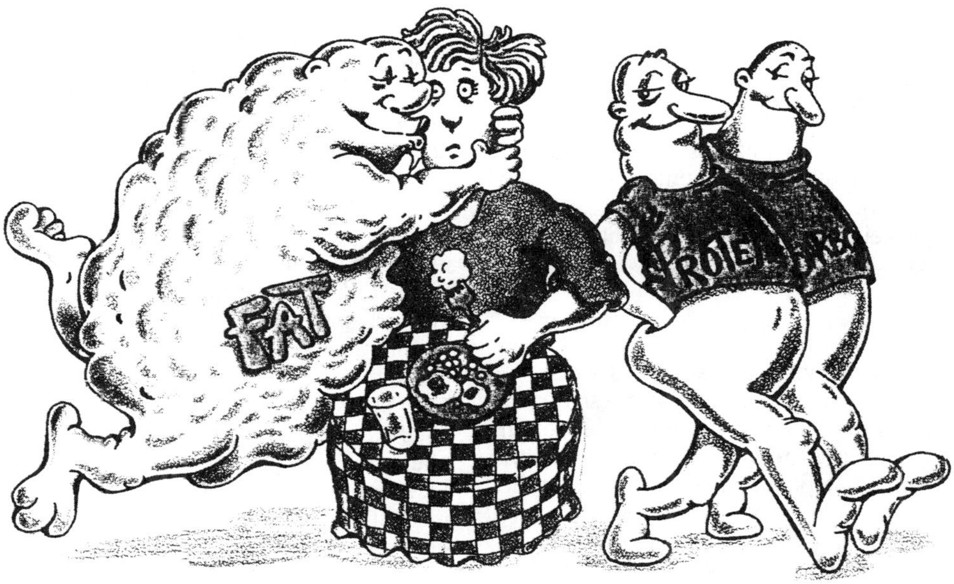

HANDLING COSTS NOT INCLUDED

Any nutritionist can rattle off the 4-7-9 rule. That is, a gram of protein or carbohydrate has 4 calories; a gram of alcohol has 7; and a gram of fat has 9. Already, fat looks bad.

But that's just the beginning. Researchers got the 4-7-9 rule by measuring the heat given off when they burned fat or protein or carbohydrate in a closed metal box. What happens in the body appears to be quite different.

"From a physical and chemical point of view, a fat calorie may equal a carbohydrate calorie, but not in humans," says Eric Jequier of the University of Lausanne in Switzerland. "There is a marked difference in the body's response to fat and carbohydrate feeding."

In fact, there are several differences. One is intuitively obvious: it's easier to turn food fat into body fat than it is to turn carbohydrate into body fat.

"In the case of carbohydrate, you pay a greater cost for handling and storage," explains Jean-Pierre Flatt of the University of Massachusetts Medical School in Worcester.

Flatt has estimated that the body's "handling" costs are:

- 3 percent to store fat as fat,
- 7 percent to store carbohydrate as carbohydrate (in a form called glycogen), and
- 23 percent to convert carbohydrate to fat.[1]

CONVERSION CATCH 22

Not only is it "expensive" to convert carbohydrates into fat, the body seems reluctant to do it.

Flatt, Jequier, and co-workers fed healthy young people 700 grams of carbohydrate—that's 2,800 calories. "The whole thing was accommodated as glycogen [carbohydrate] storage," explains Jequier. "We had to give an enormous amount of carbohydrate to see a net increase in fat deposition."

According to dieting dogma, if you eat too much carbohydrate, your body turns the excess into fat. But when they say "too much," they really *mean* it. Only when people eat massive amounts of carbohydrate does it get converted to fat.[2,3]

"Because we don't readily convert carbohydrate to fat, one has to worry separately about what happens to carbohydrate and fat," says Flatt.

That doesn't mean dieters can gorge themselves on sherbet, sodas, and other carbohydrate-rich foods and expect to lose weight. For one thing, many overweight people have problems handling carbohydrates, especially sugars. For another, you still have to eat fewer calories than you expend in order to lose weight.

CARBOHYDRATES UNDER CONTROL

The more carbohydrate you eat, the more carbohydrate you store—and the more you burn. But that's not true for fat.

Flatt fed young men a low-fat breakfast of bread, jam, and dried meat.[4] On another day, they were fed the same breakfast, with an extra 10 pats of margarine. But on the margarine day, their bodies didn't adjust by burning a greater proportion of fat.

"You have to watch out for fat calories more than carbohydrate calories, because the body maintains carbohydrate and protein balance automatically," Flatt explains. "But it doesn't control fat as well."

His co-worker, Eric Ravussin, is now at the National Institute of Diabetes and Digestive and Kidney Diseases in Phoenix. Ravussin has just completed a study on both lean and obese people that supports the earlier findings.[5]

"The body is able to cope with excess protein and carbohydrate, but not excess fat," says Ravussin.

PROGRAMMED TO BE PLUMP?

Fat's tendency to stick to the ribs (and thighs and hips) doesn't entirely explain why some people are trim and others are plump. If it did, everyone eating a typical, fat-laden American diet would have a fat-laden body.

Animal studies illustrate this point. When albino mice are fed low-fat diets, almost all stay trim.[6] The more fat (and the less carbohydrate) they're fed, the less uniform they look. Some grow fat, others stay slim—just like humans.

Clearly, genetics seems to play a role in obesity. One way genes may act is by determining how well (or how poorly) your body handles fat.

Trudy Yost of the University of Colorado Health Sciences Center in Denver has been studying women who used to be fat, but who have stayed reasonably trim for at least a few months. The formerly-obese are critical to answering the $64,000 question in obesity research: Why are these people so likely to regain their lost weight?

THE FAT LOADER

Yost and her co-workers have been looking closely at lipoprotein lipase (LPL), an enzyme that's responsible for (among other things) loading fat into adipose (fat) cells. Apparently, the LPL in adipose tissue behaves differently in formerly-obese women.

"If a normal person eats fat, the body's response is to [lower its LPL level]," says Yost. "The normal body attempts to use fat as energy before loading it into fat cells."

But when Yost gave fat to the formerly-obese women, their LPL soared far above already-high starting levels.[7] "If you present fat calories to a formerly-obese body, the first thing that happens is that the fat is packed into cells for storage," she explains. "These bodies are preferentially pulling fat calories out for storage."

Some (but not all) genetically obese animals have high LPL levels. Yost's goal is to find out what can go wrong with LPL and "fix" it. But in the meantime, she says, the only solution is to not provide the fat calories.

"We used to say that if you eat a 1,500-calorie-per-day diet, it doesn't matter if it's fat, protein, or carbohydrate. For the formerly-obese, that isn't true. Fat calories are going to be metabolized very differently than protein or carbohydrate calories."

A TASTE FOR FAT

"If it tastes good, it must be fattening." That observation may be more true for dieters than for others.

Recent studies suggest that the fatter people are, the more they prefer the taste of fat:

- When given a choice of milkshakes made with varying amounts of cream and sugar, overweight people chose fattier shakes than their lean counterparts.[8]
- Overweight people report eating no more calories than others, but more of those calories come from fat.[9]

These studies suggest that whatever makes people fat (or even the very act of trying to stay thin) also makes them crave fatty foods. But if they can fight the craving by thinking of fat—not just calories—as the enemy, it might help.

THE BOTTOM LINE

"I can tell you right now, the people in our clinic who are taught to keep fat out of their diet do better at keeping the weight off," says Elliot Danforth of the University of Vermont. "But no one will believe it unless we keep 100 people or so in a locked ward or dormitory for two-to-three years. That's a mega-expensive study."

Other researchers have made similar observations. Claude Bouchard and colleagues at Laval University in Quebec, Canada, had eight overweight women exercising five times a week for two years. The women lost weight, but then the losses leveled off—until his colleagues recommended a 20 percent low-fat diet.

"Their weight loss was spectacular," says Bouchard. "Some lost 50-to-60 pounds."

But Bouchard's women might have eaten fewer calories on the low-fat diet. The question is: will a 1,000-calorie low-fat diet lead to thinner bodies than a 1,000-calorie high-fat diet? So far, no one knows.

A low-fat diet is not a magic wand that will eradicate obesity. Clearly, genes influence your chances of tipping the scales, as does exercise. But eating less fat is also likely to help.

"If a formerly-obese woman eats 1,500 calories of fat, she's sunk," says Yost. "If she eats 200 calories of protein, 100 calories of fat, and 1,200 calories of carbohydrate, she has a chance." □

[1] Bray, G.A., *Recent Advances in Obesity Research* 2:221, 1978.
[2] *Am. J. Physiol. 246*: E62, 1984.
[3] *Am. J. Clin. Nutr. 48*: 240, 1988.
[4] *J. Clin. Invest. 76*: 1019, 1985.
[5] *Am J. Physiol. 255*: E332, 1988.
[6] *Int. J. Obes. 9*: 443, 1985.
[7] *J. Clin. Endocrinol. Metab. 67*: 259, 1988.
[8] *Physiol. Behav 35*: 617, 1985.
[9] *Am. J. Clin. Nutr. 47*: 406, 995, 1988.

Name ______________________

Section ______________________

Date ______________________

Chapter 3

QUESTIONS FOR REVIEW

1. Overweight is defined as 110 to 120 percent of ideal body weight (IBW). Obesity is defined as greater than 120 percent of IBW. Gross obesity is greater than 200 percent of IBW.

2. As weight increases, so does the occurrence of:

   a. ↑ blood press ♡ disease

   b. ↑ LDL

   c. ↑ blood glucose

   d. ↑ joint stiffness

3. The goal of dieting is to lose body fat, not muscle.

4. For the best long-term results, one should:

   a. exercise

   b. eat less cal.

   c. change habits

5. The "Yo-Yo dieting syndrome" occurs because
   wt loss slow ↓ & ↑ gain faster
   genetic

6. The "rule of 10" suggests that to lose weight slowly a female would eat 10 times her weight in kilocalories per day and a male would eat 12 times his weight.

7. Anorexia nervosa afflicts primarily young/old, males/females from poor/rich families.

8. A person might be suspected of being anorexic if she loses more than 25 percent of her body weight, or if she is less than 80% of her ideal body weight.

9. The anorexic has a distorted attitude about food and her body image

10. List 3 medical problems of anorexia nervosa.

a. amenorrhea

b. hypotension

c. bulimia

11. After nutritional supplementation, the proper treatment for anorexia nervosa is behavior ther. for the anorexic and family therapy for the family.

12. Bulimia is also called the binge / purge syndrome.

13. Purging in the bulimic may take the form of vomit or excessive use of laxatives.

14. The bulimic eats high calorie, high sugar, high-fat foods when binging.

15. Medical problems associated with excessive vomiting include:

a. esophageal rupture

b. (?) burn

c. loss tooth enamel

16. Medical problems associated with excessive laxative use include:

a. dehydration

b. mineral imbalance

c. constipation

17. Like the anorexic, the bulimic needs behavior/psychotherapy counseling.

CHAPTER 4

Dietary Carbohydrates

Carbohydrates are macronutrients that primarily provide energy in the diet. The average person in the United States consumes approximately 40 percent of his dietary kilocalories as carbohydrates. Much of this consumption is in the form of simple sugars such as sucrose. Americans eat over 125 pounds of sugar per year, per person. The United States' dietary goals are to reduce the consumption of simple sugars and increase the consumption of complex carbohydrates (starches). Total carbohydrates should be 55-60 percent of dietary kilocalories.

How much sugar do we eat?

Carbohydrates are often abbreviated CHO because carbohydrates only contain carbon, hydrogen and oxygen atoms. Two kinds of CHOs are considered in this chapter: sugars and starches (Table 4-1). Both sugars and starches contain *monosaccharides* — the simplest carbohydrate unit. The sugars, technically known as *disaccharides*, consist of two linked monosaccharides. Starches, technically known as *polysaccharides*, are long chains of monosaccharides.

Disaccharides

Disaccharides (meaning two sugars) provide kilocalories and are the major sweetening agents in the diet. Sucrose, which is table sugar, and lactose, which is the CHO found in milk, are the most common disaccharides found in foods. Most people are not aware that the sweetness of fruits and vegetables is largely due to naturally occurring sucrose. A few products such as malt and honey contain another disaccharide, maltose. The suggested relationship between sugars and various disease states will be discussed later in this chapter.

Table 4-1. Classification of carbohydrates.

Monosaccharides	Disaccharides	Polysaccharides
1. glucose	1. sucrose	1. starch (long glucose chains)
2. fructose	a. glucose	a. amylose
3. galactose	b. fructose	b. amylopectin
	2. maltose	2. cellulose
	a. glucose	
	b. glucose	
	3. lactose	
	a. glucose	
	b. galactose	

Polysaccharides

The dietary *polysaccharides* (meaning many sugars) are more commonly known as starches or fibers. *Starches,* either *amylose* or *amylopectin*, are long chains of glucose units. *Fibers,* most notably cellulose, are also long glucose chains. The difference is that humans can digest (break down) starches into individual glucose units for absorption, but humans are unable to digest fibers into smaller units for absorption. The fibers pass relatively undigested through the upper part of the intestine causing effects in the lower bowel. Potatoes, corn and rice are significant sources of starch in the diet.

Carbohydrate Digestion: Carbohydrates must be digested to their simplest monosaccharide units before they can be absorbed into the body. Each disaccharide has a specific enzyme that breaks the molecule into its individual monosaccharides. The two starches, amylose and amylopectin, also must be digested to glucose before absorption. The enzymes involved in carbohydrate digestion are listed in Table 4-2. Notice that the name of each enzyme reflects the name of the carbohydrate it digests. Sucrose is digested by sucrase, lactose by lactase, amylose by amylase, etc.

Table 4-2. Enzymes of Carbohydrate Digestion

Carbohydrate	Digestive Enzyme	End Product of Digestion
Disaccharides		
1. Sucrose	Sucr*ase*	Glucose; Fructose
2. Lactose	Lact*ase*	Glucose; Galactose
3. Maltose	Malt*ase*	Glucose; Glucose
Polysaccharides		
1. Amylose	Amyl*ase*	Glucose
2. Amylopectin	Amyl*ase*	Glucose
3. Cellulose	Not Digested by Human	Enzymes

Lactose intolerance

A genetic condition, *lactose intolerance*, exists in much of the world's population. In cultures (primarily Black and Asian) in which the adult does not traditionally consume milk products, the body has gradually lost the ability to make the enzyme lactase. In these populations lactase is present during breastfeeding in infancy but after weaning is no longer produced. In populations that have been traditionally herd keepers, such as a few African tribes and Northern Europeans, lactase is made by the body throughout life because these populations have consumed milk products throughout their lives.

When lactase is not present, the unabsorbed lactose continues into the large intestine. In the large intestine, bacteria "feed" on the lactose causing it to be broken into many components. The resulting lactose intolerance occurs 3 to 4 hours after the ingestion of milk products. Lactose intolerance is characterized by *gas production, bloating, diarrhea* and *cramps.*

How can lactose intolerance be avoided in people traditionally exhibiting these symptoms? Unfortunately, once the body stops making lactase, this ability cannot be recovered. It is not possible to adapt by increasing one's intake of milk products. Yet people who suffer from lactose intolerance can sometimes tolerate small amounts of milk products. Each individual has a different threshold at which symptoms occur.

Until recently persons severely affected by lactose intolerance were forced to avoid milk products completely. Now products are available that pre-digest lactose. These products take two forms. First, persons suffering from lactose intolerance can buy the enzyme lactase (Lact-Aid) at the drug store. About one-half hour before drinking, the enzyme is added to the milk. The enzyme breaks the lactose into glucose and galactose in the glass. When the milk is consumed, the problem no longer exists. It is also possible to buy milk directly from the supermarket in which the enzyme is predigested. These milk products have the same taste as regular milk. The only difference is that the lactose is digested before it reaches the intestine.

Glucose Metabolism: Once glucose is absorbed into the body, it goes first to the liver and then into the blood. After a meal, blood glucose levels rise. This elevation in blood glucose causes the hormone ***insulin*** to be released. Insulin is necessary to enable cells (muscle cells and fat cells) to absorb glucose from the blood. As the cells, with the help of insulin, absorb glucose, blood levels return to normal.

Diabetes

Some people are unable to control their blood glucose levels. This condition is called ***diabetes***. In one type of diabetes (Type I-juvenile-onset diabetes) the body no longer makes insulin. After a meal, a diabetic without insulin is unable to control blood glucose levels. The elevated blood glucose occurring in diabetes is called *hyperglycemia*. Diabetics need to be careful about how much carbohydrate they consume, especially their consumption of simple sugars. Simple sugars are rapidly absorbed and require a much greater amount of insulin to prevent abnormal blood glucose rises.

Diabetics often must adjust the amount of insulin they need to their dietary intakes. If the diabetic consumes complex carbohydrates, this adjustment is much easier because complex carbohydrates are more slowly digested. Some dietary fibers also slow the absorption of sugars and reduce a diabetic's insulin need.

A second type of diabetes (Type II-adult-onset diabetes) occurs in overweight adults. Unlike juvenile-onset diabetes, adult-onset diabetes is characterized by excess blood insulin levels. However, this insulin is ineffective and incapable of helping cells absorb glucose after a meal. The adult-onset diabetic, like the juvenile-onset diabetic, has elevated blood glucose levels. If the adult-onset diabetic loses weight and/or increases his exercise, his insulin often becomes more effective, resulting in more normal blood glucose levels.

In the liver, glucose has three fates. First, some glucose is used immediately for *energy*. Second, the liver stores glucose after meals as *glycogen*. The third metabolic fate of glucose is to *convert to fat any extra glucose* that is not stored as glycogen. Because the brain and other nervous tissue must use glucose from the blood for fuel, blood glucose levels cannot fall too low. Between meals the liver slowly releases glucose from the glycogen stores to keep blood glucose levels normal.

If blood glucose drops below a certain level (about 40 to 50 mg glucose per 100ml of blood), the brain stops receiving enough glucose to function properly. A low blood glucose level is called *hypoglycemia.* True hypoglycemia is rare, but when it occurs it causes listlessness and sluggishness in a person. If blood glucose levels fall too far too fast, too little fuel gets to the brain. This can cause a person to go into a coma. After the liver has stored all the glycogen possible, any *extra carbohydrate is converted to fat.*

The liver has the capacity to store enough glycogen to keep blood levels constant if a person does not eat for about 24 hours. After 24 hours of fasting, liver glycogen stores run out. In long-term fasting or starvation, the liver must synthesize new glucose. It does this by breaking down muscle and other protein sources and converting the amino acids found in those proteins to glucose. This process is called *gluconeogenesis.*

The muscle also has the capacity to store glucose as glycogen. The function of glycogen in muscle is to provide glucose to be used for energy during exercise. The harder one exercises, the more glucose is used for energy. During aerobic exercise (long-time, low-intensity) very little glucose from glycogen is used for energy by the muscle. Although the muscle metabolizes primarily fat for its energy during endurance events, there is good evidence that the duration of exercise depends on the amount of one's muscle glycogen. A person cannot continue to exercise much past the time his muscles are depleted of glycogen. Glycogen loading is used by athletes in some sports to allow the muscle to store as much glycogen as possible.

The original regimen followed to maximally increase muscle glycogen had a person eating a very low-carbohydrate, high-fat diet for 2-3 days after an intensive training bout. Research has shown that intensive exercise will deplete the exercised muscles of glycogen. About two days before the event, one switches to a high-carbohydrate diet (60-70 percent of the kilocalories as carbohydrates). This regimen increases muscle glycogen levels to almost twice the normal levels. However, one cannot undergo this regimen too often or the effect is lost. Also, while one is following this diet, he becomes nervous, irritable and often cannot sleep.

To reduce the stress that occurs with glycogen loading, the regimen has been modified. Now one trains and eats as usual, but about 3 days before the event one starts eating a very high-carbohydrate diet (70-80 percent of kilocalories as carbohydrates). This process puts almost as much glycogen into the muscle as the original regimen but is much easier for the athlete to tolerate.

How much does glycogen loading actually help one's athletic performance? For most weekend athletes it probably doesn't help very much. Glycogen stores are very rarely the limiting factor in performance except in endurance events of longer than three hours. Sometimes the technique of glycogen loading is used to offset poor training habits. An untrained athlete, even with maximal glycogen stores, will still not be competitive with the trained athlete. Even given that glycogen stores need to be maximized, most distance athletes, even world class athletes, do not consciously attempt to increase their glycogen levels. The well-trained athlete, by virtue of his training regimen, already has a greater capacity to store glycogen (or he couldn't run 15 miles, or bike 35 miles each day in training). These athletes simply increase their carbohydrate consumption and taper down their training before an event. These small changes along with the traditional pre-event high-carbohydrate spaghetti dinner work to increase the athletes' glycogen levels.

Sugar and Health: Americans consume a lot of sugar in their diets. Excessive sugar consumption has been implicated as a cause of many health problems such as diabetes, hyperactivity in children, and aggressive behavior. In most cases the data does not support these claims. But there are two cases in which sugar does contribute to health problems.

Sugars provide "empty calories".

Sugar provides "empty" calories and very few nutrients. Many people, especially women and growing children, are consuming diets that contain sub-optimal amounts of some nutrients (iron, calcium, vitamin A, etc.). The consumption of foods containing a lot of sugar makes it more difficult to consume the needed nutrients. Replace the sugar with fruits, vegetables and whole grains and the nutritional content of the diet greatly improves.

A second health problem that is caused or at least worsened by sugar consumption is poor dental health. Tooth decay is significantly increased when people consume sugar, especially sticky, solid sources of sugar. The sugar becomes trapped between a person's teeth. Bacteria in the mouth use the sugar for food, producing an acid. This acid breaks down the protective enamel coating of one's teeth. Overall tooth decay, especially in children, is greatly reduced in the United States today. This reduction is because of the programs that fluoridate the water supply. Fluoride makes teeth much stronger and less susceptible to the action of the acids produced by bacteria. The occurrence of tooth decay can be still lessened by reducing one's sugar consumption, especially between meals.

Dietary fiber

Dietary fiber: Dietary fiber is a term that encompasses all of the food components that are not digested. Dietary fibers pass through the upper intestine to the lower intestine where they cause their effects. Most of the dietary fiber found in foods is complex, indigestible carbohydrate. Cellulose, the most common dietary fiber (wood and paper are primarily cellulose), is just long chains of glucose molecules similar to starch. However, the glucose molecules are attached to each other in a way that prevents their digestion by human enzymes. The most common kinds of dietary fiber are *wheat bran, oat bran, cellulose (found primarily in vegetables)* and *pectin (found in fruits, vegetables and seeds).* Metamucil, psysillum seed, agar and guar gum are more exotic examples of dietary fibers.

Even though dietary fibers are not absorbed in the upper part of the intestinal tract, they still have a major impact on one's health.

The major effect of dietary fibers is to increase *laxation.* Dietary fibers cause laxation by *increasing fecal bulk, increasing fecal water* and *increasing the speed of intestinal transit.* Increased laxation results in larger, softer stools. Increased laxation decreases constipation and makes it easier to defecate.

Diverticulosis

The more fiber one has in his diet, the less likely he is to develop *diverticulosis*. Diverticulosis is a disease that occurs very frequently in the elderly consuming the typical low-fiber, high-fat diet of developed nations. Diverticulosis does not occur in the elderly of developing countries where high-fiber foods are eaten.

Diverticulosis is a disease of the colon. Low-fiber diets cause constipation. As a result, outpockets form in the colon of people as they age. These pockets become filled with fecal matter and often become sore and inflamed. Diverticulosis can be prevented if one eats a high-fiber diet over his lifetime. In the elderly who have already developed diverticulosis, high-fiber diets reduce the symptoms.

The only proven beneficial health effect of dietary fibers is to reduce the incidence of diverticulosis. There are other suggested health benefits of a high-fiber diet, however. First, a *high-fiber diet is by definition also a low-fat diet.* Excessive fat consumption is implicated as a causative factor in many degenerative diseases, such as cancer, heart disease, obesity and gallbladder disease. Second, the consumption of many *dietary fibers, most notably oat bran, pectin and Metamucil, causes blood cholesterol levels to decrease.* This is beneficial in reducing the risk of heart disease. Third, dietary *fibers have been hypothesized to reduce the risk of colon cancer.* Colon cancer is very rare in countries that consume high-fiber diets. However, it is also true that these same countries consume low-fat diets. Excessive fat consumption may be the cause of colon cancer, not low-fiber diets. Dietary fibers, by increasing fecal water, may act to reduce the risk of colon cancer by diluting the concentration of any carcinogen. Dietary fibers may also be protective because they speed up the rate of passage through the intestine. Thus, a potential carcinogen has less time to act on the intestinal wall before it is removed from the body.

If you want to increase your consumption of dietary fiber, increase your consumption of fruits, vegetables and whole grains. It is *not* recommended that you consume purified fiber sources. Too much purified fiber will interfere with the absorption of trace minerals, especially iron, zinc and copper, from the diet. Many people, especially women and growing children, are consuming less than optimal amounts of these trace minerals. Continual consumption of purified fiber sources may cause one to develop trace mineral deficiencies.

To summarize, you should attempt to reduce your consumption of simple carbohydrates while at the same time increasing your consumption of complex carbohydrates. This can be accomplished by increasing your intake of fruits, vegetables and whole grains. Diet changes of this nature will also increase your dietary fiber intake.

■ PICKING THE BEST CEREAL ■ WHEN INDIAN WOMEN COOK ■

Eater's Digest

BY BONNIE LIEBMAN

Sorting Out The Cereals

"Breakfast candies" aside, how do you pick a winner?

As shoppers wander down the cereal aisle, cross-eyed from reading the tiny print, many yearn for a simple answer to a simple question: Which cereal is best?

Companies make the search tougher by dropping and introducing new healthy-sounding cereals at a rapid-fire pace. Names like Just Right, Nutrific, NutriGrain, Fruit Wheats, and Mueslix seem carefully crafted to appeal to health-conscious consumers.

And appeal, they do. The $5 billion cold cereal market posted sales gains of 11 percent in 1986 (the last year for which figures are available). The average American now eats 11.3 pounds of cold cereal each year.

Picking a Winner. Even a novice can eliminate the sugar-laden Count Choculas and Apple Jacks. But "breakfast candies" aside, selecting the best cereal is still not easy, because no single product is perfect for everyone.

Bran cereals are highest in fiber, but most have added sugar or the artificial sweetener, aspartame. Other whole-grain choices, like Shredded Wheat and NutriGrain, have no added sugar, but their fiber levels are only moderate.

Then you have to consider the *type* of fiber you're getting. If your cholesterol is high, you'll want the soluble fiber found in oats. If you're more concerned about avoiding constipation and possibly colon cancer, it's the insoluble fiber in wheat bran that you'll need.

Because no one cereal meets everyone's needs, we've categorized the better cereals according to their most important features. Choose the category that best suits you. Then check the chart on page 12 for some specifics.

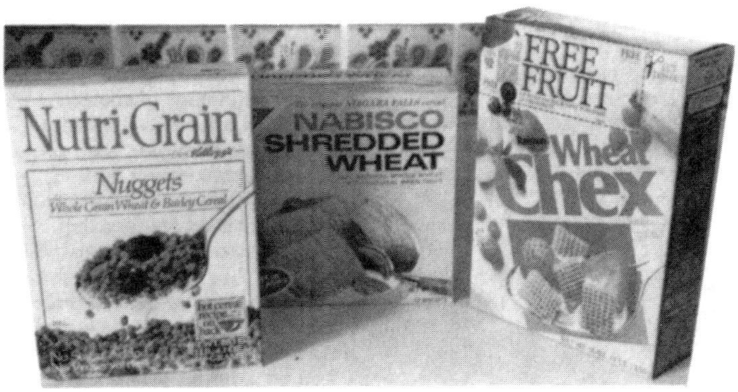

If you want fiber but little *or no sugar, choose one of these cereals.*

Highest-Fiber

What Are They? Cereals containing 10 to 13 grams of insoluble fiber from wheat bran. Most are fortified with about 25 percent of the USRDA for several vitamins and minerals.

Who Needs Them? If your goal is to prevent constipation and colon cancer, and you don't eat lots of whole-grain breads, beans, fruits, and vegetables during the rest of the day, this one's for you.

Choices:

❋ Sugar-Sweetened: All-Bran or 100% Bran contain 10 grams of fiber and just over 1 teaspoon of sugar per 1-ounce serving. That means they're about 18 percent sugar.

❋ Aspartame-Sweetened: Fiber-One and All-Bran with Extra Fiber are sweetened with aspartame instead of sugar. These cereals contain an extra 3 to 4 grams of fiber because aspartame takes up less space than sugar. Companies fill the space with more bran.

❋ Unsweetened: If you want neither aspartame nor sugar, choose a medium-fiber, low-sugar cereal (see below), and sprinkle unprocessed wheat bran on top. Each level tablespoon of unprocessed wheat bran provides 1½ grams of fiber.

Medium-Fiber, Low-Sugar

What Are They? Cereals that contain 2 to 4 grams of largely insoluble fiber from whole wheat, but have little or no added sugar.

Who Needs Them? If your goal is to prevent colon cancer and constipation, but you get some fiber from other food and you want no added sugar or aspartame, choose one of these.

Choices:

❋ Biscuits: Shredded Wheat offers no salt as well as no sugar. It isn't fortified with extra vitamins and minerals, but many people don't need an extra shot of nutrients in their cereal bowls anyway.

❋ Flakes: NutriGrain cereals and Wheaties are fortified with about 25 percent of the USRDA for several vitamins and minerals. Total is identical to Wheaties, except that the fortification levels are 100 percent. A 12-ounce box of Total also costs 58 cents more.

❋ Nuggets: NutriGrain Nuggets have twice as much fiber as Grape Nuts, and less salt to boot. Both brands are fortified with 25 percent of the USRDA for several vitamins and minerals.

Medium-Fiber, Sweetened

What Are They? Whole-grain cereals that supply 2 to 4 grams of fiber plus 1 to 3 teaspoons of sugar. Most companies won't say how much sugar comes from the dried fruit added to their cereals. We estimate that about half comes from dried fruit, the rest from refined sweeteners.

Who Needs Them? People who want some fiber, but need a few teaspoons of sugar to "make the medicine go down."

Choices:

❋ Biscuits: Like Shredded Wheat, sweetened biscuits such as Raisin or Strawberry Squares, Fruit Wheats, and Frosted Mini-Wheats have no added salt. Each has just over 1 teaspoon of sugar. Only Nabisco, maker of Fruit Wheats

Eater's Digest

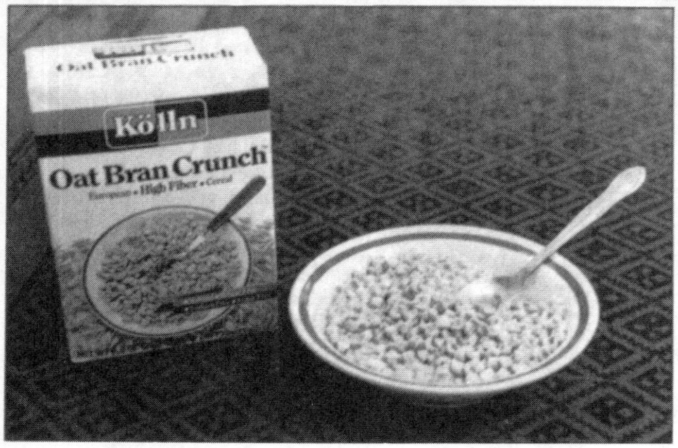

No American-made cold cereal is *high in soluble fiber, like Oat Bran Crunch, a cold cereal made in West Germany.*

cereals, was willing to reveal how *much* sugar—slightly over half—comes from fruit. Unlike Shredded Wheat, these biscuits are fortified at the usual 25-percent-of-the-USRDA level.

✱ Fruit and Flakes: Banking on Raisin Bran's popularity, cereal companies are now adding other dried fruits and/or nuts to flakes. The result is cereals such as Fruit 'n Fibre, Fruitful Bran, Nutrific, and Just Right. Each serving contains 2 to 3 teaspoons of sugar, which means the cereal is 30 to 45 percent sugar.

✱ Mixed Flakes: One of the latest trend in cereals is to mix several grains. Kellogg's Pro-Grain, for example, contains wheat, corn, and oats, plus lots of sugar (39 percent). Others, such as Grape Nuts Flakes, are lower in sugar, but fiber levels are uniformly modest, at about 2 grams per serving.

Hot and Unsweetened

What Are They? Whole-grain cereals without added salt or sugar.

Who Needs Them? People who want insoluble fiber to reduce the risk of colon cancer and constipation, but who also enjoy a hot breakfast. Or, those who want oats' soluble fiber, which lowers blood cholesterol.

So far, no American-made cold cereals have as much soluble fiber as regular oatmeal or oat bran. Oat Bran Crunch, a cold cereal from West Germany, is available in some food co-ops and natural food stores. It is high in soluble fiber, but at about $4 per pound, Oat Bran Crunch is also high in cost.

Choices:

✱ Oats: Oat bran and quick oatmeal offer soluble fiber—and no added salt, sugar, or extra vitamins or minerals.

✱ Whole Wheat: Wheatena and Ralston Hot Cereal offer *in*soluble fiber, with no added salt, sugar, vitamins, or minerals.

✱ Sweetened: Quaker Instant Oatmeals and Ralston Sun-Maid Instant cereals have fiber. But most also contain 2 to 4 teaspoons of added sugar—more than most people would spoon on at the table. Since unsweetened, unsalted Quick Oatmeal and Ralston's regular hot cereal take less than 1 minute to cook—and you can easily throw in a handful of raisins for extra sweetness—there's no reason to buy the sugared instant versions.

Last and Least

Too Much Fat. Granolas and Cracklin' Oat Bran contain

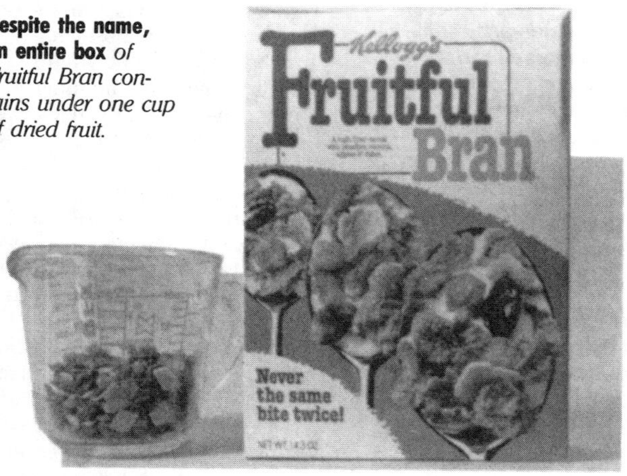

Despite the name, an entire box *of Fruitful Bran contains under one cup of dried fruit.*

Cereal Secrets

Where's the Fruit? Many cereal boxes show heaping bowls of fruit. Yet often it turns out there isn't much fruit inside. An entire box of Fruitful Bran for example, contains 1.3 ounces of fruit. That's less than one cup. Consider adding your own dried (or fresh) fruit instead.

How do you spell honey? S-u-g-a-r. Honey is no more healthful than sugar. But because honey has a better image, cereal makers use it extensively—in their product names. For example, Honey Nut Cheerios, Honey Smacks, Nut & Honey Crunch, Honey Buc Wheat Crisps, Honeycomb, Honey Graham Chex, and Honey Nut Crunch have more sugar (or corn syrup) than honey.

Fiberless Crunch. Don't assume a cereal is high in fiber just because the name sounds fibrous. Nut & Honey Crunch, Crispy Wheat 'n Raisins, Crispix, Rice Krispies, and Super Golden Crisp are low in fiber.

The Best Germ in Town. Wheat Germ is a gold mine of nutrients, from the B vitamins to vitamin E and folic acid. If you're cutting back on red meat, look no further for a rich source of iron and zinc.

The Vitamin Game. Ever read the nutrition labeling on cereal boxes? General Mills adds vitamin C to all but three of its cereals. Kellogg adds the vitamin to about two-thirds of its adult products. Post adds it to none.

Or take iron. Kellogg adds iron to all but its NutriGrain cereals. Post and General Mills add the mineral to all their products, but the levels range from 10 to 100 percent of the USRDA.

These are just a few examples of the fortification free-for-all that exists in cereal land. Manufacturers cite "current trends in eating habits" and the "nutritional needs of the American people" to explain their fortification practices. Yet it's doubtful that Kellogg has inside information showing that NutriGrain eaters need less iron.

In fact, technical feasibility and marketing strategy are what motivates many fortification decisions.

When it comes to vitamin C, for example, General Mills' Katherine Newton explains, "Most of our cereals are fortified to the 25 percent level—except those with fruit, because the moisture makes the vitamin C unstable." On the other hand, the company adds *100* percent of the USRDA for iron to Total to fill that cereal's "market niche."

Check the label if you think you need a particular nutrient. Vegetarians are one group which may benefit from cereals' extra iron and zinc. But don't get snowed by heavy-duty fortification. If you need a vitamin pill, just take one. □

Eater's Digest

about 1 teaspoon of fat, and it's often artery-clogging coconut oil. While 1 teaspoon of fat isn't much, cereals should be low in fat to leave room for foods that can't be fat-free, such as meat, poultry, and cheese.

Too Little Fiber. Five of the 10 most popular cold cereals—Corn Flakes, Rice Krispies, Honey Nut Cheerios, Frosted Flakes, and Cap'n Crunch—contain less than 2 grams of fiber. So do Cream of Wheat and Cream of Rice. These products won't hurt you, but they won't do you much good in the all-important fiber department.

One Ounce or Two? According to cereal labels, a serving of cereal is one ounce, period. Yet one ounce of the denser cereals, such as Grape Nuts, fills only one-quarter of a cup, while one ounce of the airier cereals, like Cheerios, fills one and one-quarter cups.

Indeed, government surveys show that people eat about a bowl's worth of cereal, regardless of how many ounces the bowl contains. We typically eat less than one ounce of the lighter cereals, and over two ounces of the heaviest cereals.

The chart below lists fiber and sugar levels for one ounce of cereal, but beware the "serving size" column. Assess *your* "serving size" and adjust the other numbers accordingly. □

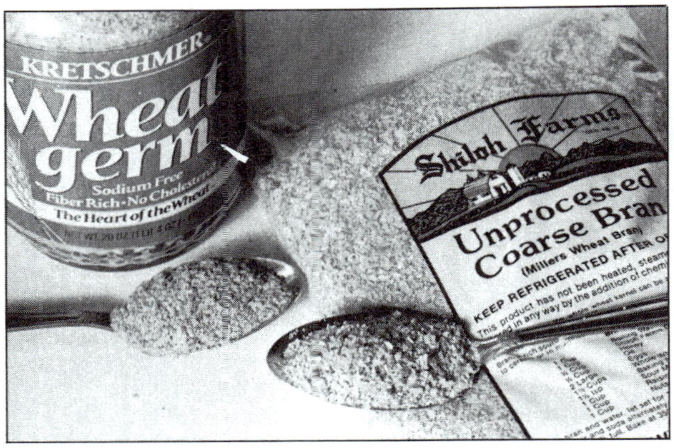

Wheat germ is a terrific source *of iron and zinc. Wheat bran is loaded with insoluble fiber.*

CEREAL SCOREBOARD

COLD CEREALS

	SERVING (1 oz)	FIBER (g)	SUGAR (%)
Highest-Fiber			
All Bran w/ Extra Fiber+	½ c	**14**	0
Fiber One+	½ c	**13**	0
100% Bran	½ c	**10**	18
All-Bran	⅓ c	**10**	18
Bran Buds	⅓ c	**10**	25
Medium-Fiber, Low-Sugar			
Shredded Wheat 'n Bran	⅔ c	**4**	0
NutriGrain Nuggets	¼ c	**4**	3‡
Wheat Chex	⅔ c	**4**	7
Wheat Germ	¼ c	**3**	0
Shredded Wheat	⅔ c	**3**	0
NutriGrain Corn	½ c	**3**	7‡
NutriGrain Wheat	⅔ c	**3**	7‡
Wheaties	1 c	**2**	11
Cheerios	1¼ c	**2**	3
Grape Nuts	¼ c	**2**	11‡
Medium-Fiber, Sweetened			
Nutrific Oatmeal Flakes	¾ c	**6**	32
Bran Chex	⅔ c	**5**	18
Bran Flakes	⅔ c	**5**	18
Mueslix Bran	⅓ c	**4**	39
Kellogg's Raisin Bran	½ c	**4**	32
Fruitful Bran	⅔ c	**4**	28
Fruit & Fibre	½ c	**4**	46
Post Raisin Bran	½ c	**4**	53
Fruit Wheats	½ c	**3**	18
Frosted Mini-Wheats	4	**3**	21
Strawberry or Raisin Squares	½ c	**3**	18
Amazin' Raisin Bran	1 c	**3**	42
Raisin Nut Bran	½ c	**3**	25
Bran Muffin Crisp	⅔ c	**3**	32
Mueslix Five Grain	⅓ c	**3**	42
Grape Nuts Flakes	⅞ c	**2**	18

COLD CEREALS, CONT.

	SERVING (1 oz)	FIBER (g)	SUGAR (%)
Just Right, Nugget & Flakes	⅔ c	**2**	18
Pro-Grain	¾ c	**2**	39
Low-Fiber			
Corn Chex	1 c	**1**	11
Rice Chex	1⅛ c	**0.5**	7
Kellogg's Corn Flakes	1 c	**1**	7
Product 19	1 c	**1**	11
Nut 'n Honey Crunch	⅔ c	**0**	32
Crispy Wheat 'n Raisins	¾ c	**0**	35
Crispix	1 c	**0**	11
Rice Krispies	1 c	**0**	11
Special K	1 c	**0**	11
Honey Nut Cheerios	¾ c	**0**	35
High-Fat			
Cracklin' Oat Bran	½ c	**5**	25
Quaker 100% Natural	¼ c	**2**	25
C.W. Post Family Style	¼ c	**1**	25
Nature Valley Granola	⅓ c	**1.3**	21

HOT CEREALS#

	SERVING (1 oz)	FIBER (g)	SUGAR (%)
Medium-Fiber			
Ralston High-Fiber Cereal	⅔ c	**5**	0
Wheatena	5/6 c	**4.5**	0
Oat Bran	⅔ c	**4***	0
Oatmeal, Quick	⅔ c	**3***	0
Low-Fiber			
Cream of Wheat	¾ c	**1**	0
Cream of Rice	¾ c	**0**	0

Note: All nutrient data comes from the manufacturers.

*A good source of *soluble* fiber, which can help lower blood cholesterol. Most other high-fiber cereals are rich in insoluble fiber, which helps prevent constipation, diverticulosis, and possibly colon cancer.

+Sweetened with aspartame (Nutrasweet).

#Serving size based on cooked cereal.

‡Naturally occurring sugar in grains and malt flavoring.

Name ______________________

Section ______________________

Date ______________________

Chapter 4

QUESTIONS FOR REVIEW

1. What are two U.S. dietary goals related to the consumption of carbohydrates?

   a.

   b.

2. A disaccharide consists of 2 monosaccharides.

   A polysaccharide consists of many chains monosaccharides.

3. Two examples of disaccharides are sucrose and lactose maltose.
   Amylopectins is an example of a polysaccharide.

4. Dietary fiber is a polysaccharide that is/is not digested.

5. Carbohydrates are digested by enzymes that have the same name as the carbohydrate but end in ase instead of -ose.

6. Lactose intolerance occurs because certain peoples cannot digest lactose because their body does not have the enzyme lactase. A lactose deficiency is characterized by gas/bloating, flatulence and cramps.

7. Diverticulosis occurs because people do not eat enough dietary fiber.

8. The three metabolic fates of glucose in the body are:

   a.

   b.

   c.

9. Glycogen loading is used to increase the glycogen content of the muscle/liver. (Select one)

10. Dietary fibers increase laxation. Laxation is:

a. ↑ stool size

b. ↑ " H_2O

c. ↑ transit rate

11. Two other diseases that increasing your dietary fiber may protect you against are:

a. colon cancer

b. ♡ diseases

CHAPTER 5

Dietary Fats

Lipid is the technical term for fat.

Dietary fats are the most calorie-dense of the nutrients from which we derive energy. A gram of fat provides 9 kcals, while a gram of protein or a gram of carbohydrate provides only 4 kcals each. This means that 100 grams (not quite 4 ounces) of pure fat, such as butter, contains 900 kcals while 100 grams of sugar contains 400 kcals. It is often stated that carbohydrates are fattening. Relative to fats this is not true. A baked potato, which is predominantly carbohydrate with a small amount of protein, is not particularly fattening, especially if one considers the nutrients obtained from a baked potato per kcal. However, when butter or sour cream, both high-fat products, is added to the baked potato, the caloric content increases dramatically.

A baked potato is not fattening.

Dietary fat consumption

Dietary Fat Consumption Patterns and Recommendations: Americans consume approximately 37-42 percent of their dietary kilocalories from lipids or fats. Most of this intake is in the form of hidden fats, fats that are not readily apparent in the foods. While it is easy to see the fat that surrounds meat or the fat in raw hamburger, most fat is not so easily observed. For instance, in a glass of whole milk (3.3% fat) approximately 48% of the kilocalories come from lipids. In contrast, a glass of low-fat milk (2.0% fat) has 33% of the kilocalories as fat. Skim milk has less than 5% of its calories derived from lipids. Table 5-1 provides the percentage of calories obtained from the fat portion of some popular foods. The kcals from fats in chocolate chip cookies are surprising to most people: 33% of total calories. Also, most people are very surprised to find out that 81% of the kilocalories in hot dogs and 85% of the kilocalories in bologna are from fats.

Table 5-1. Percentage of kilocalories from fat in selected foods.

Food	Kcals/serving	Kcals from Fat
Milk, whole	160 (1 cup)	48%
Milk, low-fat	120 (1 cup)	33%
Milk, skim	80 (1 cup)	<5%
Cheese, cheddar	115 (1 oz.)	77%
Cookie, chocolate chip	200 (4 cookies)	35%
Hot Dog	170 (1 link)	81%
Bologna	85 (1 slice)	86%
Big Mac (McDonalds)	563	53%
French Fries (McDonalds)	220 (regular)	47%
Green Beans, cooked	30 (1 cup)	<2%

As previously stated, in the United States lipids account for approximately 40-45% of dietary calories. While the percentage of kcal from fats has slightly decreased in recent years, it is still higher than most experts would recommend. It is thought that a reduction in dietary fats, besides reducing the dietary caloric content, will be beneficial because a low-fat diet reduces the risk of heart disease and perhaps reduces the risk of cancer. While it is advisable to reduce fat consumption as much as possible, the recommended dietary goals (Table 5-2) are to reduce fat intake to 30% of dietary kilocalories. Even this intake, given the nature of the typical American diet, will be difficult but not impossible to reach. A motivated individual could reach this goal by carefully limiting processed, convenience and fast foods.

Table 5-2. Recommended dietary changes related to fat consumption.

1. Reduce total dietary energy from 45% of kcals to 30% or less.
2. Adjust energy consumption to 10% of kcals each from saturated, monounsaturated and polyunsaturated fats.
3. Limit dietary cholesterol to less than 300 mg/day.

The triglycerides

Besides reducing total fat intake, it is also important to be aware of the different fats in our diets and their health implications. The fats generally consumed in the diet are *saturated fats* (found in animal products), *monounsaturated fats* (found in olive oil), and *polyunsaturated fats* (found in other vegetable oils). As a group these fats are known as *triglycerides*. The chemical differences between each fat will be discussed later in this chapter. Ideally, people should consume equal amounts of saturated fats, monounsaturated fats and polyunsaturated fats, with no more than 10% of one's kcals from any fat source.

Currently, the American public consumes too much saturated fat, causing blood cholesterol to increase and increasing the risk of heart disease. We can offset the cholesterol-raising effects of saturated fats by increasing polyunsaturated fats (vegetable oils) in our diets. However, evidence is accumulating that intakes of polyunsaturated fats over time, above the recommended 10%, may increase a person's risks for developing other diseases such as gallstones or even certain cancers. Thus, one should not try to offset the negative effects of a high-saturated-fat diet by increasing one's intake of polyunsaturated fat. It is much more beneficial to decrease total fat consumption, especially saturated fats. By decreasing total fat consumption, it is possible to consume equal amounts (10% of kcals) of each group of fats.

Cholesterol

A final recommendation is to limit one's intake of dietary cholesterol. Cholesterol is also a dietary fat, but one that has a much different structure than triglycerides (saturated, monounsaturated and polyunsaturated fats). People with high blood levels of cholesterol have an increased risk for developing heart disease. There is good evidence that many people with high blood cholesterol would benefit by reducing their dietary cholesterol intake. However, there is still controversy about this dietary recommendation because dietary cholesterol intake has no effect on blood cholesterol levels in some people. If one has elevated blood cholesterol levels, it is sound advice to limit one's intake of eggs, organ meats (liver, kidney), dairy products and fatty meat products that are especially high in cholesterol.

Chemistry of lipids

Chemistry of lipids: The main lipids in the diet are called *triglycerides* (Figure 5-1). Triglycerides consist of three fatty acids attached to one glycerol unit — thus the term tri (three) glyceride (glycerol). It is the fatty acids that determine whether the triglyceride is a saturated, monounsaturated or polyunsaturated fat. Fatty acids are long chains of carbon atoms with a COOH (acid) group at the end. Each carbon atom, besides being attached to other carbon atoms, also binds hydrogen atoms. A *saturated fatty acid* is one in which all of the carbon atoms are "saturated" or filled up with hydrogen. A *monounsaturated fatty acid* is one in which the hydrogen atoms between two carbon atoms are missing, creating a single double bond. Thus, monounsaturated means one double bond. *Polyunsaturated fatty acids* have two or more double bonds on the carbon chain.

Figure 5-1. Structure of triglyceride, and saturated, monounsaturated and polyunsaturated fatty acids.

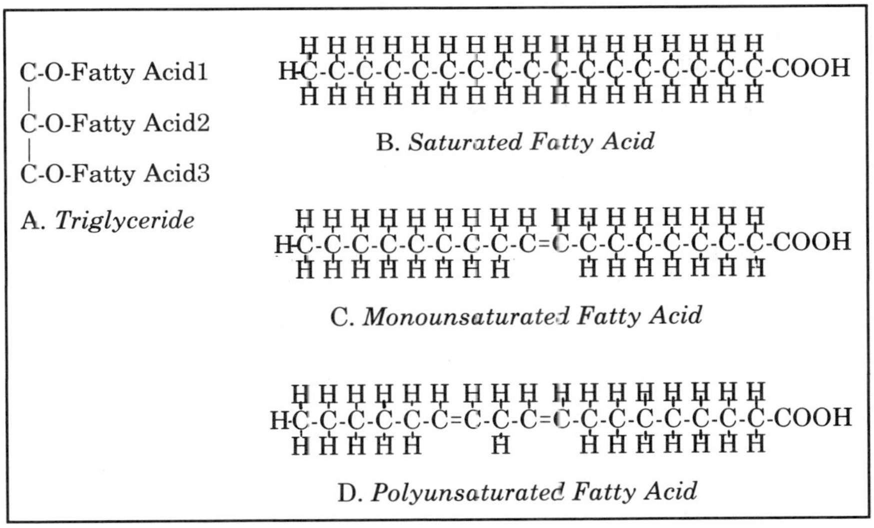

The fats one eats are triglycerides consisting of saturated, monounsaturated, and polyunsaturated fatty acids. These fats have different chemical characteristics depending on which fatty acids they contain. The more unsaturated a fat is, the more liquid it is at room temperature. Saturated fats are solids at room temperature. Triglycerides consisting of predominantly saturated fatty acids are solids at room temperature, and thus called dietary "fats." Examples of dietary fats are lard, butter, beef tallow and the solid fat in cuts of meat. Triglycerides that are liquid at room temperature are called dietary "oils." Vegetable oils and salad oils are examples of

Fats vs. oils

triglycerides that contain polyunsaturated fats. Olive oil is a specific example of a food that contains large amounts of monounsaturated fats. It is a liquid at room temperature.

Figure 5-2. Comparison of dietary fats

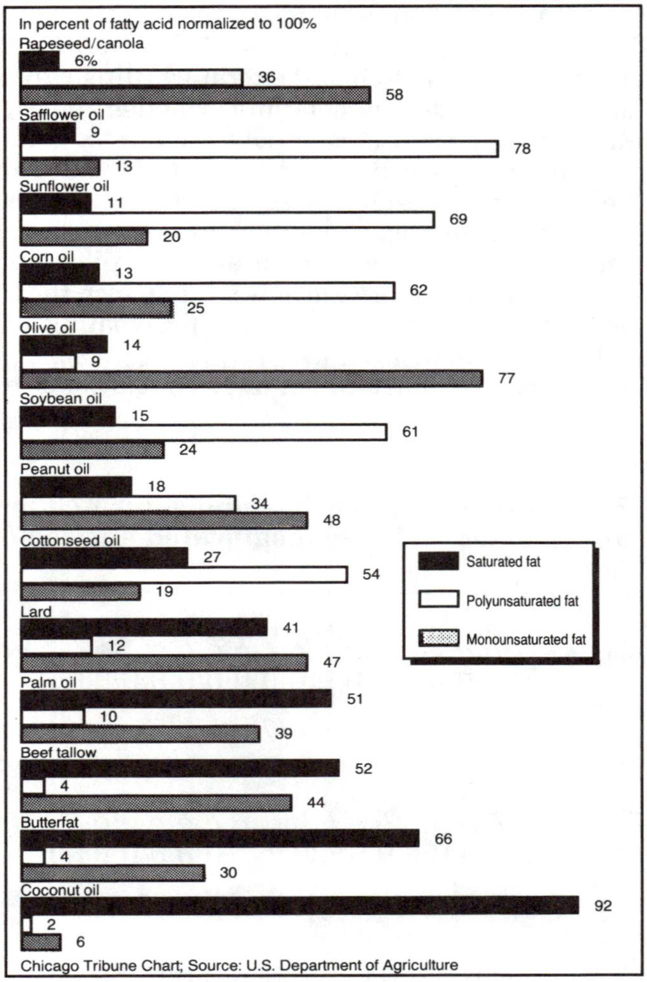

Hydrogenated fats

Natural fats and oils are often modified or chemically altered by the food industry to improve food products. You should be familiar with some of the terms on food labels that describe these fat modifications. The most common term that occurs on food labels is *hydrogenated* or sometimes *partially hydrogenated*. Polyunsaturated fats tend to be very unstable and very susceptible to becoming rancid. Food processors hydrogenate fats by adding hydrogen to the molecule, thus eliminating some of the double bonds. This makes the fat much more like a saturated fat, increasing its melting point (making the fat more solid at room temperature) and decreasing spoilage by rancidity. Many margarines are partially hydrogenated so that the vegetable oils they contain will be solid enough that they can be molded into squares. Margarines that come as liquids in squeeze bottles have been much less hydrogenated than those that are packaged as sticks.

Besides being very liquid, polyunsaturated fats are also very susceptible to reacting with oxygen (oxidation). When a fat reacts with oxygen, it is called rancidity. The use of polyunsaturated fats in foods only occurs because food manufacturers also use ***antioxidants***. Antioxidants protect the double bonds of fats from reacting with oxygen, thus increasing the shelf life of a product (the time a product remains good). For instance, a bottle of vegetable oil opened to the air would only take about two days to become rancid without antioxidants. With the antioxidants in the salad oil, the product would remain viable for one month or more. Some common antioxidants that you may see on food labels are BHT, BHA, propyl gallate, and vitamin E.

Another term often encountered on food labels is ***emulsifier***. An emulsifier is a chemical that allows fats and water to mix, and to remain mixed. Without the use of emulsifiers many of the foods we take for granted could not be produced. For instance, mayonnaise, salad dressings, and margarine could not be produced without the use of emulsifiers. But you may say — I make mayonnaise at home and I do not use an emulsifier. In fact, you use one of nature's best emulsifiers. When you add the egg yolk to make the mayonnaise, this yolk contains a natural emulsifier called lecithin. Lecithin and other emulsifiers work by coating the small droplets of fat in a food product. This coating is charged, causing the charged fat droplets to repel each other.

Lipid Digestion: As in food systems, dietary fats and the water in your body do not readily mix. This means that your body has had to adapt in order to digest, transport and store fats. Basically, the human body is about 65-70% water. Your blood is water-based as are the digestive fluids. Thus, the body has developed its own emulsification systems to keep lipids in small discrete particles. Without this system, the fat from your diet could not be broken down for digestion and could not be transported throughout the body without "sludging" up your bloodstream.

As you eat, food in your stomach sends a message to your gallbladder telling it to eject a substance called *bile* into your intestine. Bile, made by the liver and stored in the gallbladder, is needed to emulsify dietary fats into small particles. Only when dietary fat is emulsified can it be digested. ***Lipase,*** an enzyme that digests lipids (named as are the enzymes that digest carbohydrates), breaks triglycerides into fatty acids and glycerol. Free fatty acids and glycerol can be absorbed into the intestinal cells; the whole triglyceride molecule cannot.

Bile is necessary to break fat into small particles (emulsified) so that lipase can work. A person who cannot make bile cannot digest fats. A person who has had his gallbladder removed cannot store bile. This person must eat very small, low-fat meals. If he eats too much fat at one meal, without sufficient storage of bile he is unable to digest all the fat in that meal. Undigested fat cannot be absorbed. The fat then continues through the intestine, and is excreted in the feces. High fat in the feces is called ***steatorrhea***. Besides the unpleasantness of steatorrhea, failure to digest and absorb fats can also mean a failure to absorb fat-soluble vitamins and, if the condition continues long enough, can lead to vitamin deficiencies.

Lipid Absorption and Transport: Once fatty acids and glycerol (the products of fat digestion) have been absorbed into the intestinal cell, triglycerides are re-synthesized from these components. However, the body still has to transport this water-insoluble fat through the lymph and blood to the various tissues of the body. The body does this by creating an emulsified particle called a lipoprotein. A lipoprotein (Table 5-3) is a small molecule in which fat (either triglyceride or cholesterol) is surrounded by emulsifiers (proteins or phospholipids). The protein and phospholipids form charges on the outside of the lipoprotein, repelling other lipoproteins. This charge allows the lipoprotein to move through the water-based blood without "sludging" up. In the intestinal cells a lipoprotein called a chylomicron is made to allow the transport of dietary fats. *Chylomicrons are lipoproteins that carry dietary fats from intestinal cells, through the blood, to tissues.*

Table 5-3. Classification of lipoproteins.

Lipoprotein	Main Function
Chylomicron	Transport dietary fats from intestine to tissue
Very Low Density (VLDL)	Transport fats made in liver to tissues for storage
Low Density (LDL)	Transport cholesterol to tissues for storage
High Density (HDL)	Transport cholesterol from tissues to the liver for excretion

When we eat excess kilocalories as dietary protein or carbohydrate, the body converts them to fat in the liver. This endogenously synthesized fat then has to be transported to the adipose tissue (fat stores) for storage. Again, the body does this by making a lipoprotein

VLDL

called a *very low-density lipoprotein (VLDL). VLDL transports fats made in the liver to the adipose tissue for storage.*

LDL

The body also makes lipoproteins to transport cholesterol. *Low-density lipoproteins (LDL)* transport cholesterol through the blood to peripheral tissues for storage. Most people are not aware that cholesterol is needed by the body to form cell membranes. In fact, much more cholesterol is made in the body than is consumed in our diets. Thus, LDL is needed to carry this cholesterol through the blood.

HDL

Another lipoprotein, *high-density lipoprotein (HDL),* takes cholesterol from peripheral tissues and carries it to the liver where it is excreted. These two systems for carrying cholesterol, LDL and HDL, work in opposition to each other.

Cholesterol and Heart Disease: Many studies in both animals and humans have shown that as blood cholesterol levels increase, the risk for developing heart disease increases. When a person's blood cholesterol is determined by a physician, the value (total cholesterol) includes both the LDL-cholesterol and the HDL-cholesterol. The current recommendations suggest that an adult's desirable total cholesterol levels should be less than 200 mg/dl (mg/dl are the units that express the concentration of cholesterol in one's blood). At blood cholesterol levels below 200 mg/dl, there is little risk of developing heart disease. As long as one's total cholesterol value is normal —less than 200 mg/dl — the different lipoprotein cholesterol levels are not as important. This is because at low total cholesterol levels the LDL-cholesterol (bad cholesterol) is also generally low.

Cholesterol limits

Figure 5-3. Narrowing of an artery due to cholesterol accumulation.

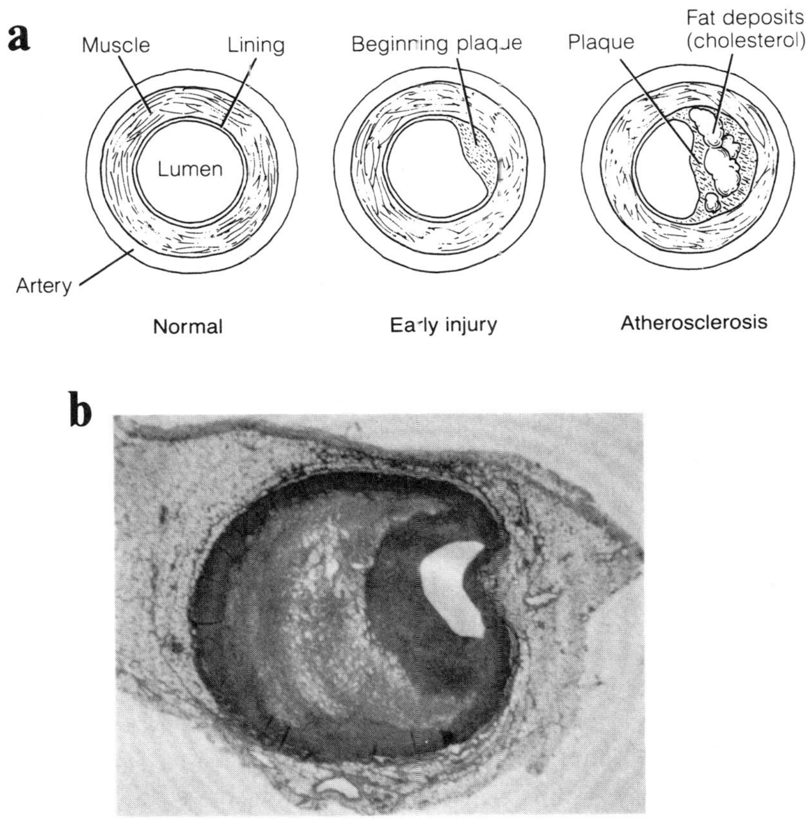

(a) This figure shows the progression of atherosclerosis in the cross-section of an artery. (b) This micrograph shows a human artery that is almost completely blocked.

From: *Nutrition for Living*, 2nd Edition, J.L. Christian, J.L. Greger, Benjamin Cummings Publishing Co.

A blood cholesterol level between 200 and 239 mg/dl is considered borderline-high, while a cholesterol level above 240 mg/dl is considered high. A second cholesterol test should be undertaken in anyone that has a cholesterol value above 200 mg/dl. If the second test confirms the first test, then a complete lipid profile should be done. This lipid profile will determine total cholesterol, HDL-cholesterol and triglyceride concentrations.

"Good" and "bad" cholesterol

LDL-cholesterol is the "bad" cholesterol. The higher one's LDL-cholesterol, the greater the risk for developing heart disease. Elevated LDL-cholesterol levels mean that more cholesterol is available to be deposited into arteries. HDL-cholesterol, on the other hand, is the "good" cholesterol. The greater one's HDL-cholesterol, the less risk one has for developing heart disease. Increasing one's HDL-cholesterol levels causes cholesterol to be taken from arteries and carried to the liver.

Heart disease (Atherosclerosis)

Heart disease (Atherosclerosis) is an accumulation of cholesterol in the arteries of the heart (Figure 5-3). The three major risk factors in developing heart disease are *elevated blood cholesterol levels*, *high blood pressure* and *cigarette smoking*. As cholesterol accumulates in the cells of the artery, the artery narrows until eventually blood can no longer pass through the opening. When this happens a myocardial infarction (heart attack) occurs. Each of the risk factors makes it easier for cholesterol to be deposited into the arteries. High blood pressure and cigarette smoking destroy the protective layer of cells on the surface of the artery that prevents cholesterol deposition. The higher one's blood cholesterol, the more likely it is that cholesterol will be deposited in the arterial cells. Having one risk factor increases the risk of developing heart disease to two times that of a person not exhibiting any risk factors. But if one is at risk for two factors, the risk increases to at least four times that of someone not exhibiting any risk factors. Someone who has elevated cholesterol, high blood pressure, and smokes will have greater than 16 times the probability of having a heart attack than someone without any risk factors.

HDL-cholesterol protects the body from developing heart disease because it removes cholesterol from the arterial wall and transports this cholesterol to the liver. People trying to reduce total cholesterol should also try to increase HDL-cholesterol relative to LDL-cholesterol.

Diet change to affect cholesterol levels

The easiest way to lower blood LDL-cholesterol levels is by changing one's diet. Some effective dietary changes that lower LDL-cholesterol levels in most people are listed in Table 5-4. In persons with borderline-high cholesterol levels (200-239 mg/dl), the first treatment is to change the diet as described in Table 5-4. Often these dietary modifications can result in a 15-20 percent decrease in blood cholesterol levels. In persons with high cholesterol levels (above 240 mg/dl), dietary changes alone may not lower blood cholesterol levels enough. Often, diet modifications are combined with drug therapy to effectively reduce one's blood cholesterol. Research has shown that for every 1 mg/dl decrease in blood cholesterol levels there is a 2 percent decrease in heart disease. So even moderate decreases in blood cholesterol concentrations can reduce the incidence of heart disease. HDL-cholesterol levels do not respond to diet as dramatically as do LDL-cholesterol levels. However, some lifestyle and dietary changes can increase HDL-cholesterol levels.

The best way to minimize heart disease development is by moderate lifestyle changes. One should not smoke or should quit smoking if one already smokes. Blood pressure should be monitored, and attempts should be made to bring it under control (many of the same lifestyle changes for heart disease are used in the initial treatment of high blood pressure). One should try to exercise as frequently as possible. Exercise, including walking, should be undertaken as frequently as possible but at least three times a week. Moderate diet changes can also significantly decrease one's risk for heart disease. To reduce the fat in the diet drink low-fat or skim milk. Substitute fresh fruits and vegetables as often as possible for high-calorie, high-fat products. The inclusion of more fresh fruits and vegetables will not only reduce the fat content of one's diet but will also change the type of fat consumed to a more unsaturated fat, and beneficially increase the fiber content of the diet. Remember, a healthy diet does not have to exclude any foods. Just eat a variety of foods, and try to moderate your consumption of high-fat, calorically dense foods.

Table 5-4. Factors that reduce total (LDL) cholesterol, and increase HDL-cholesterol levels in the blood.

Factors that lower total cholesterol levels

1. Decrease total dietary fat consumption
2. Increase dietary polyunsaturated and monounsaturated fat intake
3. Replace animal protein with vegetable protein
4. Increase dietary fiber consumption
5. Reduce dietary cholesterol intake
6. Lower dietary minerals intake, such as chromium, and a low zinc/copper ratio

Factors that increase HDL-cholesterol levels

1. Females have higher levels than males
2. Exercise increases HDL-cholesterol
3. Moderate alcohol consumption may increase HDL-cholesterol
4. Some dietary fibers may increase HDL-cholesterol
5. Some minerals, most notably chromium, may increase HDL-cholesterol

Fish oils

One recent fad therapy to protect against heart attacks is the use of *fish oil capsules*. Some evidence exists that the ingestion of fish oils prevents the occurrence of heart attacks in Eskimos even though they eat a very high-fat diet. The nutrition community is divided about whether fish oils, extracted and given in capsule form, offer any protection against heart disease. The proper way to obtain fish oils is by including fish in one's diet at least three times per week. To see an effect with fish oil capsules, many capsules must be consumed. Besides being expensive, some side effects have been observed as fish oil capsule consumption increased: fishy breath, allergies, vitamin A toxicity, and in some cases, excess cholesterol in the capsules. Again, this is a case where one should get his nutrition from the supermarket, not the drugstore. Since we really do not know what the long-term effects of fish oils in concentrated form are and its benefits are questionable, increase the consumption of fish in your diet.

In summary, moderate lifestyle changes can significantly decrease your chances of having a heart attack even if your blood cholesterol levels are genetically high. Do not smoke, keep your blood pressure under control and watch your diet. Try to eat less fat by eating more cereals, fresh vegetables and fruits. Try to exercise moderately at least three times per week. While these lifestyle modifications may not completely prevent heart attacks, they can significantly lessen the risk.

The Mistaken "Cholesterol Myth"

The national effort to lower cholesterol is unjustified, wasteful, and dangerous, charges Thomas J. Moore in *Heart Failure*.

The former Washington correspondent for the Knight-Ridder newspapers argues that a small cadre of researchers, armed with weak evidence and inaccurate laboratory tests, and egged on by the major drug companies, has scared tens of millions of people into believing that their blood cholesterol levels are dangerously high. Because of this, Moore charges, we are spending billions of dollars each year seeking treatment for a non-existent "affliction."

To someone not familiar with the volumes of scientific research on diet and heart disease, Moore's conclusions seem to make sense. And, if you've ever dreamed of bacon and eggs while contemplating the bowl of oatmeal on your breakfast table, you probably *want* to believe him.

That might explain why excerpts from the book, published (as "The Cholesterol Myth") in the September issue of *The Atlantic*, made headlines.

But the headlines—and Moore—are wrong. There is compelling evidence that a cholesterol-lowering diet can drastically reduce your risk of heart disease. If anything, that same diet is also likely to lower, not raise, your risk of colon cancer and stroke, not to mention obesity.

Heart Failure tells only half the story. It whines about what was *wrong* with the research that is used to justify the national program to lower cholesterol. But it ignores what was *right* about that research. More importantly, it overlooks (or misinterprets) a mountain of crucial evidence.

Here are five of the major points Moore makes, and why they are wrong or misleading.

1. *Only one out of seven people can expect to lower cholesterol by more than ten percent through diet. The most the rest of the population can achieve is a five to six percent reduction.*

This simply isn't true. Moore confuses *how much* diet can lower cholesterol with *how well* people stick to a cholesterol-lowering diet.

"If people change their diets, their cholesterol levels will drop. If they don't change their diets much, their cholesterol won't drop much," says Frank Sacks, of Harvard Medical School.

When researchers made absolutely sure healthy people were eating cholesterol-lowering diets (by keeping them in the hospital), blood cholesterol levels dropped 20 to 25 percent.

That, says Sacks, is what most of us can expect from a cholesterol-lowering diet . . . if we stay on it.

And even people who choose their own food can expect more than a five to six percent fall in cholesterol, says Basil Rifkind, of the National Heart, Lung and Blood Institute (NHLBI).

"Many different studies in free-living populations have shown a 10 to 15 percent reduction in cholesterol with changes in diet," he says. The Surgeon General, in his 1988 report, "Nutrition and Health," agreed.

So how did Moore conclude that diet could only lower cholesterol by five to six percent? He did it by misinterpreting the results of four research studies.

In fact, three of the four studies were not fair tests of diet's effect on cholesterol.

For example, in MRFIT (Multiple Risk Factor Intervention Trial), many of the participants were taking blood-pressure-lowering drugs . . . drugs that *raise* cholesterol levels, counteracting the cholesterol-lowering diet.

In the fourth study, the Diet-Heart Study, cholesterol levels dropped, as expected, by about 10 percent. Moore discounts the study because researchers did not include volunteers who were overweight or who were unlikely to follow the diet. But that doesn't mean diet *wouldn't* lower their cholesterol . . . if they stuck to it.

One more thing: Moore cites the study as evidence that only one in seven people "respond" to diet with at least a ten percent drop in cholesterol. In fact, 70 percent responded when their meals were prepared for them by dietitians, and 54 percent responded when they prepared their own cholesterol-lowering meals.

2. *Despite research that took ten years and cost more than $300 million, there is no evidence that lowering your cholesterol will lengthen your life.*

The studies Moore cites to make his case didn't show that lowering cholesterol would lengthen lives because they weren't designed to. Instead, they were designed to show that lowering cholesterol would prevent fatal and non-fatal heart attacks.

"You would need three to four times as many people or two to three times the length of time to show a drop in total mortality," explains Ron Goor, the co-author of *Eater's Choice* and the former coordinator of the National Cholesterol Education Program.

"Anyone who stops worrying about cholesterol could be ... dead wrong."

The reason you would need more time or more people is that, compared to a lifetime, even "long-term" studies are short.

"Trials like MRFIT are conducted in middle-aged men who are already highly diseased with cancer, gallstones, and diabetes—all consequences of a bad diet," explains William Connor, of Oregon Health Sciences University. "How long can you expect to extend the life of these people with an intervention started so late in life? To show prolonged life, we need to start much earlier."

Harvard's Frank Sacks agrees. "If you wait long enough, you will probably see a decrease in total mortality."

And, in fact, that's just what is now beginning to happen. As researchers follow the progress of the men who participated in the large trials, they are starting to see that those who lowered their cholesterol are dying off at a slower rate.

For example, some 15 years after the formal end of the Coronary Drug Project, people who lowered their cholesterol by taking large doses of niacin, a B-vitamin, had an 11 percent lower death rate.

Other studies that show a decrease in total mortality include the 102-month follow-up of the Oslo Diet/Smoking Study, the Stockholm Ischemic Heart Disease Project, and the long-term follow-up of MRFIT, according to reports presented at recent conferences.

Moore argues that mortality is the whole ballgame. "What difference does it make what they write on your death certificate?" he has asked in radio interviews.

But avoiding a *nonfatal* heart attack isn't trivial. "I'd rather drop dead of a heart attack at 85 than survive a serious one in middle age," says Henry McGill, of the University of Texas Health Science Center in San Antonio.

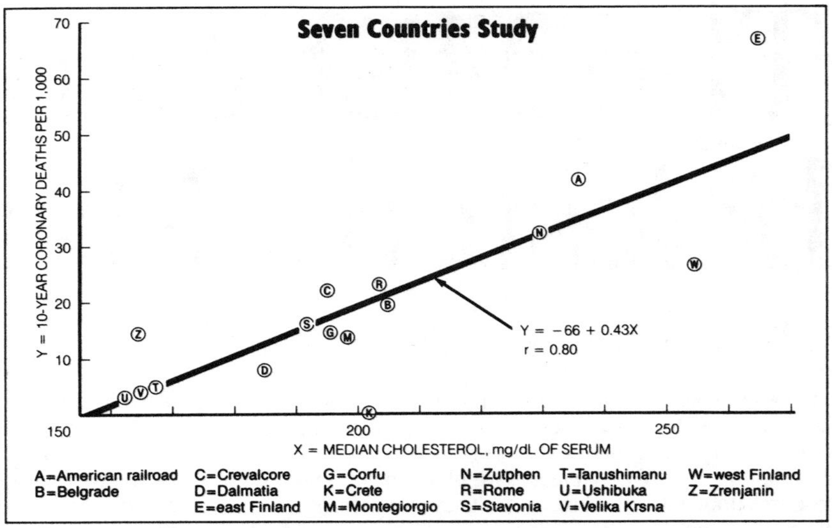

In this landmark epidemiological study, *conducted in the 1960's, populations with higher blood cholesterol levels clearly suffered more deaths from coronary heart disease.*

3. *The studies designed to show that lowering cholesterol prevents heart attacks have been failures.*

By focusing on length of life, Moore misses the more important point: Lowering cholesterol *does* reduce the risk of heart attacks—both fatal and non-fatal.

"It's amazing that people in middle-age, exposed to high cholesterol levels most of their lives, can change their risk of coronary heart disease over a four to five year period," says Richard Shekelle, of the University of Texas Health Science Center in Houston. "Four to five years is a relatively short period of time, compared to the 40 to 50 years preceding it."

Moore dismisses these studies out of hand. Instead, he plays up what he calls the "failure" of the CPPT and MRFIT.

■ MRFIT (Multiple Risk Factor Intervention Trial). More than 6,000 middle-aged men were encouraged to lower their cholesterol through modest changes in diet, reduce their blood pressure (through medication, if necessary), and stop smoking. After six years of treatment, they had no fewer fatal and nonfatal heart attacks than another 6,000 men in the "non-treatment" group.

That's what was reported in 1982, and that's what Moore makes such a big deal over. But consider this: researchers decided it would be unethical to deny treatment to the "non-treatment" group.

So these people were referred back to their private doctors, who were sent yearly reports on their patients' cholesterol, blood pressure, and other risk factors.

Not surprisingly, heart attack rates in both the "treatment" and "non-treatment" groups were much lower than expected. But without a difference *between* the groups, the study couldn't prove that lowering cholesterol prevents heart attacks.

"In the case of MRFIT, some people have mistakenly said diet had very little effect," says Shekelle. "The ['non-treatment'] group consisted of many conscientious, motivated individuals who also changed their diets and quit smoking, just like the treatment group," he adds.

Even so, in 1988, when researchers looked back at how the participants in MRFIT had fared over the years, they found that the "treatment" group is indeed living longer—and suffering fewer deaths from heart disease—than the "non-treatment" group.

Moore never mentions this . . . and a good reporter would have.

"He didn't check with the investigators, and that's a flaw in his research," says William Castelli, director of the Framingham Heart Study.

■ CPPT (Coronary Primary Prevention Trial). This ten-year trial looked at the ability of a drug (cholestyramine) to lower cholesterol. As expected, the drug-treated group had fewer fatal and nonfatal heart attacks than the control group. But Moore

"There is compelling evidence that a cholesterol-lowering diet can drastically reduce your risk of heart disease."

charges that the results were statistically significant only because the researchers used the wrong statistical test—called the one-tailed test.

Wrong again.

In fact, the alternative, a "two-tailed" test, should have been used only if researchers thought the drug might *increase* the incidence of heart attacks (which it didn't).

"All previous trials and animal studies pointed toward a benefit with cholesterol-lowering, so it was appropriate to use a one-tailed test," says Ron Goor.

Also, Moore fails to mention that those CPPT participants who faithfully took their cholestyramine for at least four years (no mean feat) reduced their cholesterol levels by more than 25 percent, and lowered their risk of coronary heart disease by 49 percent.

Moore not only misinterprets MRFIT and the CPPT, he makes an even bigger mistake: He dismisses the massive evidence showing that populations who eat cholesterol-lowering diets have fewer heart attacks. These *epidemiological* studies "provide important evidence because they show the effect of diet over a lifetime," says Shekelle.

And these studies have yielded impressive results that link lower cholesterol levels with reduced risk of heart disease.

"In observational studies of large populations," says Henry Blackburn, of the University of Minnesota, "for every difference of one percent in average cholesterol levels, there is a three percent difference in the risk of coronary heart disease."

4. *People with low cholesterol have higher rates of colon cancer and stroke.*

Cancer. At least in some studies, people with low cholesterol levels (below 180) are more likely to have colon cancer. That's all Moore needed to label colon cancer one of "the dangers of lower cholesterol." But once again, he misses key evidence.

■ If low cholesterol levels caused colon cancer, countries with low cholesterol would have high colon cancer rates. In fact, the opposite is true.

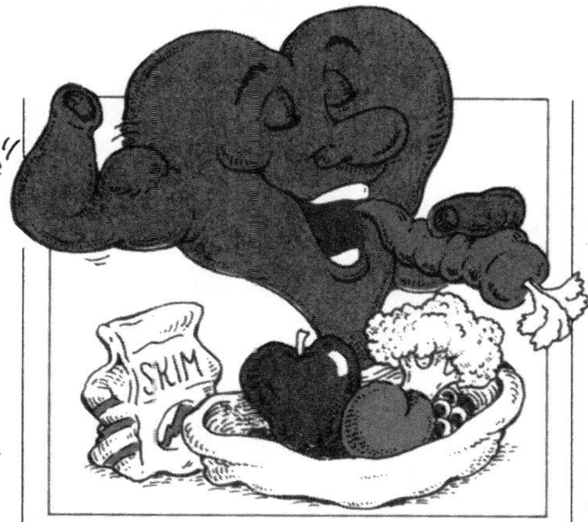

"In Japan, where cholesterol levels are low, the incidence of colon and breast cancer is lower than in the U.S.," says Oregon's William Connor.

Even in the U.S., low cholesterol is associated with low cancer rates. Seventh Day Adventists, who follow vegetarian diets, have lower cholesterol levels.

"Studies done on Seventh Day Adventists show that the men live five years longer, the women live three years longer, and both have less than half our colon cancer rate and one-tenth our heart attack rate," says Framingham's William Castelli.

Animal studies also show that the less fat, the less colon cancer. "Low-fat diets *protect* you from breast and colon cancer," says Ron Goor.

■ The studies showing a cholesterol-cancer link were too small to be considered "good evidence," according to epidemiologist Richard Peto, of Oxford University.

"You don't get this relationship in large studies," he explains. "When a Kaiser Permanente study followed 160,000 people, the relationship between low cholesterol and colon cancer just disappeared." Two other large studies, done in Honolulu and Paris, also found no link.

■ Even if people with low cholesterol levels did have higher rates of colon cancer, "there is no evidence that lowering [blood] cholesterol causes cancer," says the National Cancer Institute, in response to Moore's charges.

"To date, no cholesterol-lowering diet has caused cancer," says Oregon's Connor.

■ Most experts think that low cholesterol is the *result*, not the *cause*, of colon cancer.

"When you have cancer," explains Connor, "food intake decreases, metabolism changes, and cholesterol falls." Metabolism may also change in people whose cancer hasn't yet been detected, adds the NHLBI's Basil Rifkind.

Stroke. The second "danger" of low cholesterol, says Moore, is stroke.

His evidence? A study showing that in parts of rural Japan where cholesterol levels were below 180, "the rates of stroke were two to three times higher than areas with higher cholesterol levels."

But Moore fails to mention two points:

■ The Japanese suffer high rates of stroke caused by high blood pressure alone.

"It's hypertension that's causing the strokes," says William Connor. "The high blood pressure blows out the arteries."

Connor adds that in the U.S., this kind of "hemorrhagic" stroke isn't very common. "Here, the majority of strokes are due to the narrowing of blood vessels, which is a byproduct of a diet high in cholesterol and fat."

In other words, rather than cause strokes, a cholesterol-lowering diet helps prevent the strokes Americans suffer from most.

■ When researchers looked at Japanese people who live in large cities (as opposed to Moore's "rural" population), they saw the effects of an "Americanized" diet.

"Over the last 30 years fat intake has doubled and cholesterol levels have increased," says Framingham's William Castelli. At the same time, "the kinds of strokes have been changing from those that are the result of high blood pressure to those that are caused by both blocked arteries *and* high blood pressure."

Not surprisingly, Castelli adds, "in those same areas, coronary heart disease rates have quadrupled."

5. *A relationship between high cholesterol and heart disease cannot be found among the elderly, who suffer from a majority of heart attack deaths.*

Four out of five heart attack *deaths* occur in people over 65. But 45 percent of all heart *attacks* occur in younger people. That's why most studies involve

"Moore's assessment of the information on diet and cholesterol bears no relationship to reality."

middle-aged men.

"People need to remember that when this research started in the 1950's, the average 40-year-old male had a 20 percent chance of developing coronary heart disease before age 60," says Shekelle.

"Preventing disability and death from cardiovascular disease in middle-age; that's what this is all about."

Nevertheless, a new NHLBI study will also look at the cholesterol-heart disease link in older people. And there's reason to think it will find one.

When Moore says that cholesterol is *not* a reliable predictor of heart disease among the elderly, he cites Framingham. This study—which began in 1948 and is still going on—has monitored the health of thousands of residents of a city near Boston—and has provided researchers with much of what they know about the risk factors for heart disease.

But, says William Castelli, who directs the Framingham Study, "Moore simply doesn't understand the data that has come out of Framingham."

"Even 15 years ago, the data showed that high LDL ["bad"] cholesterol and low HDL ["good"] cholesterol were risk factors in the elderly," says Castelli. "And during the last five years," he adds, "newer data show that high *total* cholesterol is also a risk factor.

"Not only is high cholesterol related to heart disease in the elderly. If anything, cholesterol is even more dangerous to the elderly than to younger people, because the older you get, the higher the heart attack rate."

And a good reporter would have discovered that, says Castelli. "Moore never called me to ask about the Framingham Study."

The Bottom Line

"Moore's assessment of the scientific information on diet and cholesterol bears no relationship to reality. He doesn't understand the huge mass of evidence," says Harvard's Frank Sacks.

It's clear that Moore overlooked large bodies of that evidence.

For example, says Oregon's William Connor, "he completely ignored the ani-

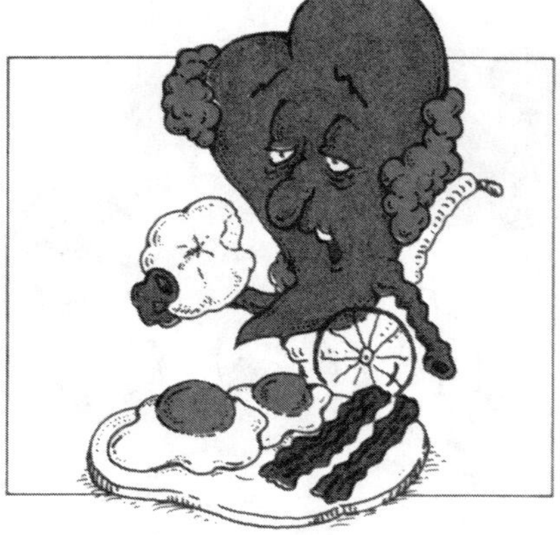

mal evidence. To produce heart disease in animals, you feed them a bad diet."

Worse yet, Moore missed the Cholesterol Lowering Atherosclerosis Study (CLAS).

In the past, the only way researchers could actually look into clogged arteries was to perform autopsies. But new technologies allowed the CLAS scientists to examine human arteries in the living.

At last, they would be able to see if lowering cholesterol could arrest or reverse the clogging process.

Beginning in 1979, a CLAS team took a group of men who had undergone coronary bypass surgery and, through diet and drugs, got them to lower their cholesterol by 26 percent. After two years, "the progression of atherosclerosis was stopped in 40 percent of the people," says Ron Goor.

What's more, the arteries of another 16 percent of the men who had lowered their cholesterol were actually in better shape than when the study began.

Missing this research is bad enough. But Moore virtually ignores the entire field of epidemiology—the study of different populations. Yet that evidence is far more important than the intervention trials Moore bases his case on.

"Laboratory and epidemiological studies should provide about 80 percent of the evidence," says Oxford University's Richard Peto. "The trials simply add a little extra."

The University of Minnesota's Henry Blackburn agrees. "MRFIT and CPPT probably didn't even need to be done. The [epidemiological, clinical, and animal] data were strong enough for public health action."

Public health action. Moore criticizes the massive cholesterol screening and treatment program recommended by the National Cholesterol Education Program. But his comments show that he doesn't understand public health strategies for fighting illness.

When a disease strikes one out of every four members of a large population, you don't try to track down and treat each potential victim. Instead, you change the environment that promotes the illness.

And when it comes to heart disease, a big part of that environment is diet.

As for the absolute proof Moore seeks, what evidence does he have that the current, high-fat American diet is best? How many will die prematurely while waiting for multi-million-dollar, decade-long studies to end? Why waste those lives and dollars?

And what would Moore replace the National Cholesterol Education Program with?

"For most of the people most of the time," he writes, "the advice of [Los Angeles cardiologist] Eliot Corday may be helpful. 'Cholesterol should be checked *only* if there are sound clinical indications,'"

"It's preposterous to wait that long," counters Framingham's William Castelli. "Sound clinical indications is just doctors' double-talk for 'you're already doomed.' By the time there are sound clinical indications, you're already having symptoms, and you've already developed heart disease."

The bottom line is clear: Studies of populations indicate that we could wipe out heart disease—which kills a half-million Americans each year—by changing the nation's diet.

"Last year there were 1.5 million heart attacks in the U.S.," says Castelli. "If we lowered the population's cholesterol by nine percent [from 210 to 191, for example], we'd have 300,000 fewer heart attacks."

And isn't that what it's all about? □

References available upon request.

Name ______________________

Section ______________________

Date ______________________

Chapter 5
QUESTIONS FOR REVIEW

1. Americans consume about 40 per cent of their kilocalories as fat. It is recommended that they only consume 30 per cent.

2. Name the three types of fatty acids and a source for each. Also name the number of double bonds in each fatty acid.

	Fatty Acid	Source	Double Bonds
a.	saturated	meat + dairy	
b.	monounsaturated	olive + canola oil	
c.	Polyunsaturated	veg, corn, soybean oil	

3. A triglyceride contains 3 fatty acids.

4. Fats are solid at room temperature while oils are liquids at room temperature.

5. The addition of hydrogens to a fatty acid during processing is called hydrogenation.

6. Bile acids help emulsfies a fat so that it can be digested by the enzyme lipase.

7. Name the four lipoproteins.

   a. VLDL

   b. LDL

   c. HDL

   d. chylomicrons

8. Name the three major risk factors for developing heart disease.

   a. plaque formation (narrow artery)

   b. HDL (↑)

   c. chollestrolle

9. For the lowest risk one's blood cholesterol level should be below ________ mg/dl.

10. The technical name for heart disease is atherosclerosis.

11. The high LDL/HDL cholesterol increases the risk of heart disease, while high LDL/HDL cholesterol decreases the risk.

12. List three dietary ingredients which lower blood cholesterol levels.

a. PUFA + mono fats

b. fiber (oat bran - pectins)

veg

c.

minerals

13. List three factors that increase blood HDL cholesterol.

a. gender

b. exercise

alcohol - modern

c.

no steroids

CHAPTER 6

Dietary Proteins

How much protein do you need? Most Americans consume well in excess of their requirement (RDA) for dietary protein. Yet, a misconception exists that for certain activities such as intense exercise or weightlifting, the need for protein is greater than the RDA. This chapter will explain what proteins are, why they are needed by the body, and how different proteins meet this need.

Proteins consist of individual units called *amino acids*. The basic structure of an amino acid is shown in Figure 6-1. Each amino acid has an amine group (NH_2) on one side of a central carbon atom and an acid group (COOH) on the other side, thus the name amino acid. In foods, there are twenty-two different amino acids; each has the same basic structure, differing only in one side (R) group. The different R groups, which can vary from a single hydrogen atom to complex molecules, make each amino acid unique.

Proteins are amino acids.

Figure 6-1. General structure of an amino acid.

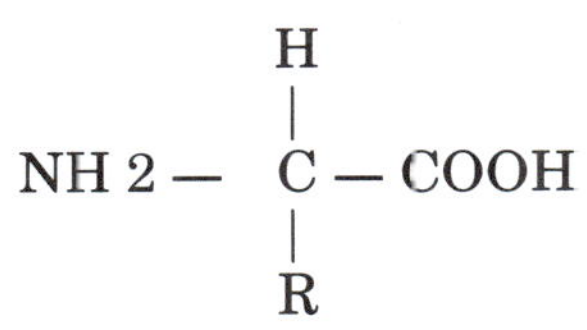

Proteins are made in the foods we eat and in our bodies by linking one amino acid to another. The amine group of one amino acid is attached to the acid group of a second amino acid in a chain-like fashion. A third amino acid is then attached, and so on, until hundreds of thousands of amino acids are linked into a protein.

Figure 6-2. Protein synthesis; linking of amino acids.

$$AA_1 + AA_2 \rightarrow AA_1 - AA_2$$
$$AA_1 - AA_2 + AA_3 \rightarrow A_1 - AA_2 - AA_3$$
$$AA_1 - AA_2 - AA_3 + AA_n \rightarrow \text{Protein}$$

Think of twenty-two different color plastic snap beads and all the different combinations that could be used to make up a chain. Chicken meat has a different texture from beef because the combination of amino acids is different.

Eight are essential amino acids

The reason that we must eat dietary proteins is to get the amino acids necessary to make proteins in our body. Of the twenty-two different amino acids found in our foods, eight are called *essential amino acids.* Essential amino acids are those amino acids that cannot be made in the body. Given the right materials our body is capable of making fourteen of the twenty-two amino acids found in foods; the eight essential amino acids cannot be made by the body and must be obtained from foods. Therefore, the functions of proteins from our diet are two-fold: 1) to provide the eight essential amino acids needed by our body, and 2) to provide the non-essential amino acids or materials for the body to make the non-essential amino acids.

When we eat proteins, we are really just eating sources of amino acids. We actually could survive very nicely by consuming the amino acids individually in the right amounts each day. However, except in patients who are fed parenterally (tube-fed) in a hospital, amino acids are only found in the proteins of our foods. The digestion of proteins in our body consists of the unlinking of each amino acid from the protein chain. After the amino acids are absorbed, they are deposited in the liver or muscle in an *amino acid pool* to be available for protein synthesis in the body.

After we eat, the body is in an *anabolic* state. This means that the body is ready to synthesize new proteins. The genetic material of the body, DNA, provides the "blueprint" for protein synthesis. That is, DNA provides the information about which amino acids are needed and in what order to synthesize a protein. For instance, if the body wanted to synthesize the protein insulin, a message from DNA would tell the order in which the amino acids would be linked. The body would get each amino acid as it was needed from the amino acid pool and add it to the protein chain until insulin was synthesized. As long as all of the amino acids are present in the amino acid pool, protein synthesis will continue. However, if one amino acid needed to make insulin is not in the amino acid pool when the body needs it, synthesis of insulin will stop. It is important, then, that all the amino acids be present in the right amounts when proteins are being made.

The ability of food to supply the proper mix of essential amino acids is a measure of that food's *protein quality.* A *complete protein* is one that supplies all the essential amino acids in the proper amounts needed for protein synthesis. Complete protein sources are eggs, milk, meat, cheeses, fish and poultry. A complete protein source, such as egg protein, if fed as the only dietary protein source (obviously not something that one commonly does in the United States) would both *support growth* in a young growing child and *maintain* an adult's protein stores.

Partially complete protein sources provide all of the essential amino acids in the proper amounts except one. This amino acid, in the protein in limited amounts, is called the *limiting amino acid*. Vegetables, legumes (seeds), and grains (rice, corn, wheat) are all examples of partially complete protein sources. However, each of these protein sources has a different limiting amino acid. For example, vegetables have a different limiting amino acid than grains (although all grains have the same limiting amino acid). A partially complete protein will *not support growth* in a growing child but will *maintain* an adult's protein stores. Making new protein in a growing animal that is increasing its protein stores takes more and better-quality protein than maintaining the protein already present in an adult. An adult who is fed just one partially complete protein would be able to maintain his protein status, but a child fed the same protein source would show signs of protein deficiencies. In the adult, the limiting amino acid would be present in sufficient quantities to replace tissue already in place, but enough of the limiting amino acid would not be available to make more tissue in a growing child.

Incomplete proteins

The last category of protein quality is *incomplete proteins*. These proteins are completely lacking one of the essential amino acids. As such, incomplete proteins are neither able to support growth in the young nor to maintain protein in the adult. An example of an incomplete protein is *gelatin*.

Kwashiorkor

Around the world protein deficiencies occur because the diet in many developing countries (especially in Africa, the Caribbean and Central America) is limited to one staple or main protein source. In these countries a protein deficiency called *kwashiorkor* develops in children consuming these diets. (Figure 6-3). Kwashiorkor is a term meaning "first-second." The first child born to a family is breast-fed (good quality protein) until a second child is born (usually 2-3 years later). The second child is now breast-fed, while the first child starts to eat the low-protein corn or taro diet. Because the child is receiving sufficient calories but not enough quality protein, a severe protein deficiency develops. Kwashiorkor is characterized by *edema* (water accumulation in the tissues resulting in swollen bellies and swollen limbs), *scaly skin, decreased immunity* and a *decreased intelligence* if the child survives. Kwashiorkor develops when adequate calories are present but the diet contains limited protein. The deficiency disease has become better understood since the mid 1960s and steps have been taken to try to prevent or lessen its occurrence (such as providing better protein sources to these people). However, politics or an inability to deliver good quality protein to where it is needed often prevents us from overcoming this problem.

Marasmus

Contrasting kwashiorkor is the more prevalent protein-energy malnutrition deficiency called *marasmus*. Marasmus, (starvation) affects young and old alike. Unfortunately, even though we grow enough food worldwide to feed everyone, we cannot, for economic, social or political reasons, always make that food available to the people that most need it.

In the United States, kwashiorkor-like symptoms have been observed in children of strict macrobiotic vegetarians. *Macrobiotic vegetarians* limit their diet to a few grain products. In adult macrobiotic vegetarians these grain products have enough of the limiting amino acids to meet their protein needs. However, in children of

Figure 6-3. Photographs of marasmus and kwashiorkor.
(From *Nutrition Today*, vol. 24, Jan. 1989)

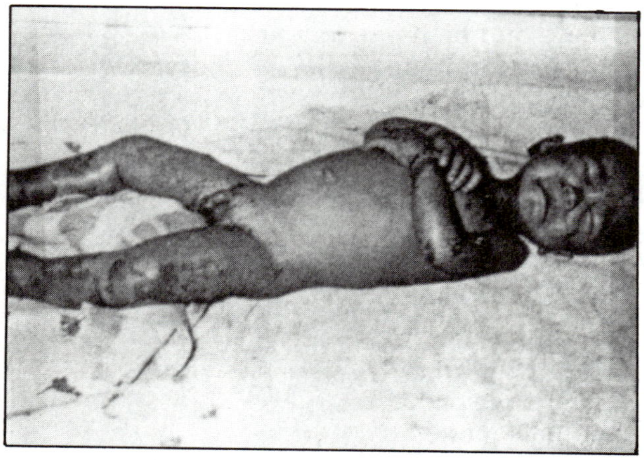

Kwashiorkor

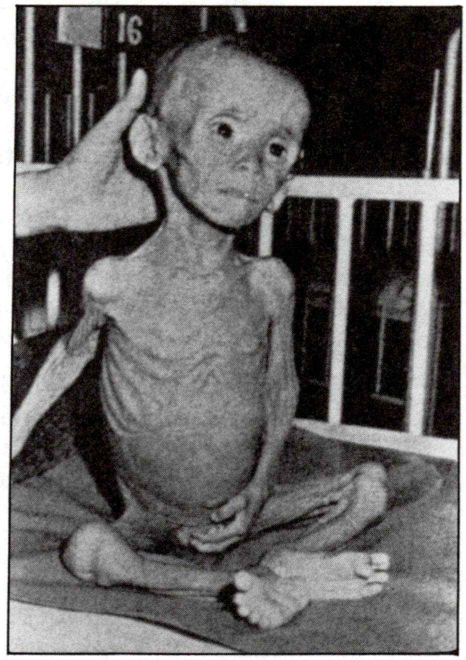

Marasmus

strict macrobiotic vegetarians, the protein sources are too limited to provide all the necessary essential amino acids. Thus, in the United States, a country in which the average person consumes over twice his requirement for protein, kwashiorkor symptoms have been observed.

Other vegetarian groups generally do not have to worry about protein quality. The *lacto-ovo vegetarian* (eats milk products and eggs) is already consuming complete protein sources. The true vegetarian who does not eat any animal products, called a *vegan,* generally is aware of protein-quality concepts. Vegans need to eat *complementary protein sources* at each meal. Complementary proteins are protein sources eaten together in which the two proteins provide the amino acid the other lacks. These complementary proteins, such as red beans and rice, must be eaten at the same meal to achieve the complementary effect.

The concept of complementary proteins is illustrated in Figure 6-4. Protein A is limiting in AA_3, whereas protein B is limiting in AA_4. Neither protein by itself is complete. When the proteins are consumed together at the same meal, each protein provides an amino acid the other lacks (panel C). Thus the proteins are complementary.

Figure 6-4. Complementary Proteins

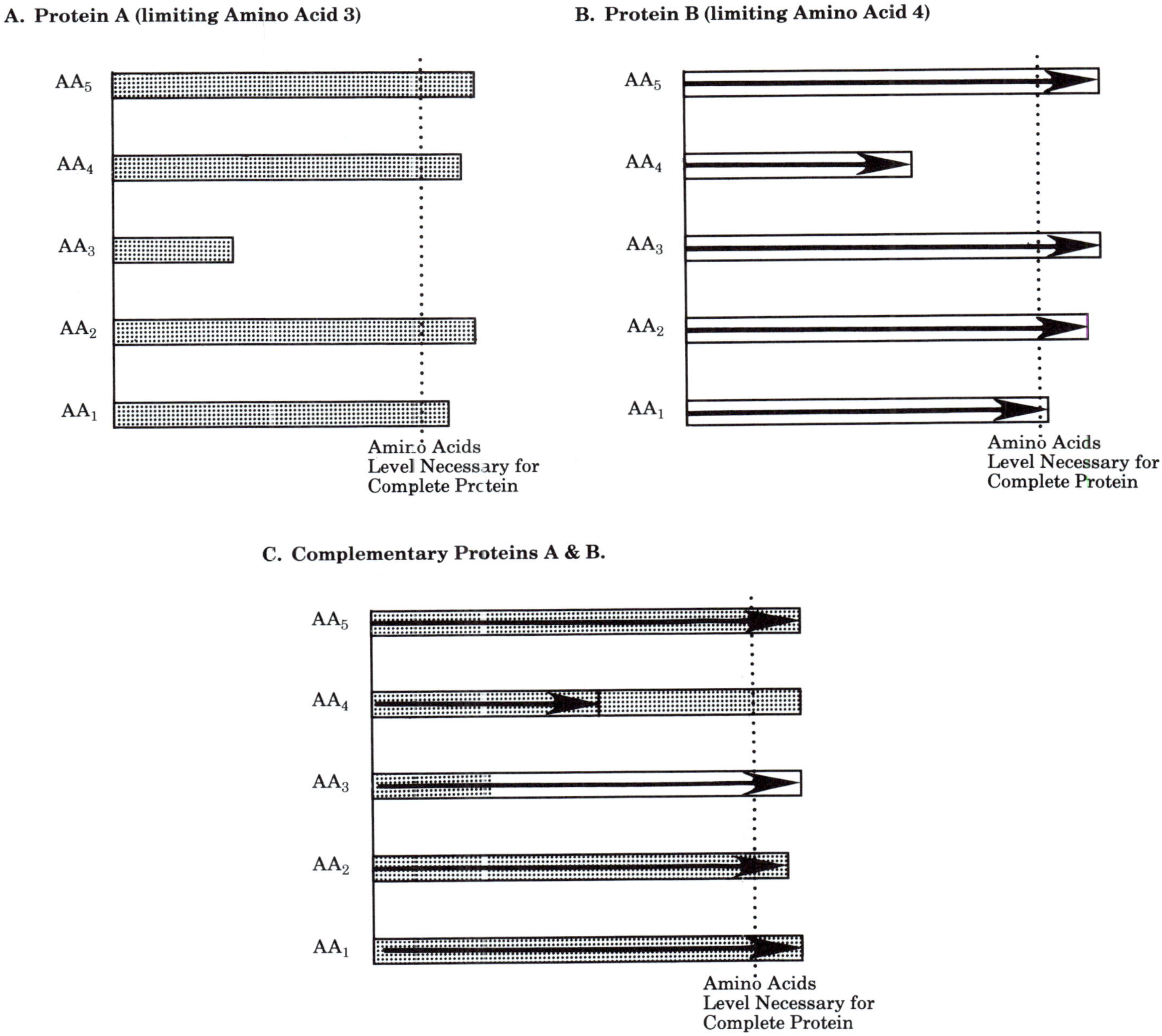

Protein requirements

Protein Requirements: How much protein does one need to consume each day in order to meet the body's needs for amino acids? Studies done over many years have concluded that the requirement (RDA) for protein in healthy adults is 0.75 grams of protein per kg of weight. Men and women have the same protein needs. This means that the 70 kg reference man needs about 52 grams of protein per day, whereas the 56 kg reference woman needs about 42 grams of protein per day. Two eggs, two pieces of toast and a glass of milk for breakfast supply over 25 g of high-quality protein — about one half of a person's need per day. A large hamburger with cheese also provides 25 to 30 grams of protein; again approximately one half of the average person's need. Studies show that the average male consumes between 110-120 grams of protein per day and the average female consumes 80-90 grams of protein per day.

The body uses dietary protein to synthesize new proteins. Proteins made in the body serve many functions. They *provide structure by forming muscles and connective tissue*. They *regulate body functions as hormones and enzymes*. Proteins help the body *regulate fluid and pH (acid base) balances*. Proteins are needed to allow one's *immune system* to function properly.

Protein conversion

If one's needs are more than met by one's protein intake, what happens to the extra protein that is eaten each day? Once the body synthesizes any protein it needs after each meal, some of the excess amino acids are *metabolized for energy,* but most of these amino acids are broken down and *converted to fat*. The body has little capacity to store amino acids. This is why complementary proteins must be consumed together to be effective. As the body produces a certain protein, if an amino acid is not present, the body stops making that protein. The other amino acids used in making that protein cannot be stored until the limiting amino acid is obtained from the next meal. The body assumes that the amino acids that are not used because of the unavailability of the limiting amino acid are surplus and breaks them down, converting the excess to fat.

Other than conversion to fat, there appears to be little evidence that excessive intake of proteins is harmful. Many years ago it was thought that excessive protein intakes would damage one's kidneys, but this has been disproven in healthy people. (However, people with kidney failure must severely limit their protein intake.) Recent evidence suggests that excessive protein intake may increase the rate of calcium loss from the body. This may accelerate the course of *osteoporosis* (discussed in Chapter 9), especially in women already at risk for osteoporosis. Luckily, there appears to be no acute toxic effect of protein overconsumption in healthy people.

A question often asked about protein requirements is: do I have an increased protein need if I am an intense athlete or weightlifter? *All* of the evidence currently available conclusively shows that athletes more than meet their protein needs from their dietary protein intake. In some intense training and weightlifting regimens, an athlete's protein needs may be slightly increased over the average person's. However all *controlled scientific* studies suggest that RDA for this small elite group can be more than met with 1.2 g protein per kg body weight. This means an intensively training person weighing 100 kg would have a requirement of 120 grams of protein per day. This value is within the average that most adult men consume daily.

A common misconception is that the intensive athlete and/or weightlifter needs much larger intakes of proteins in order to stimulate protein metabolism. It is often suggested at health clubs or gyms that a serious weightlifter should consume 2.2 grams of protein per kg of body weight to stimulate muscle formation. The rationale is that one should "flood" the system with amino acids in order to maximize muscle synthesis. There is no evidence that these large intakes increase muscle mass or the ease with which one builds muscle. Hard work stimulates muscle formation, not excessive dietary protein intake.

Amino acid intakes

Amino Acid Intakes: Recent trends in protein nutrition center around the consumption of individual amino acids. In the past, one consumed foods that contained a mixture of amino acids. It was difficult to isolate the effect of an individual amino acid because all foods contain a mix that is eaten, digested and absorbed at the same time. However, with the recent advent and popularity of nutrient supplementation, one is able to purchase and consume almost any dosage of any amino acid. This has led to much nutrition misinformation about the effects of these isolated amino acids in the body. Unfortunately, the misinformation has spread faster than the nutrition community's capability to investigate each claim. One claim currently in vogue is that consumption of the amino acids ornithine, arginine and lysine will stimulate growth hormone release. To date, we do not have enough scientific, valid information to evaluate some claims about the effects of individual amino acids on metabolism. However, it still appears to be true that if something "seems too good to be true," or promises a response with little or no effort, then that supplement is probably worthless.

Overdosing On PROTEIN

BY ELAINE BLUME

The Great Protein Myth has its roots in the last century, and has been perpetuated by well-meaning nutritionists and self-serving industries. According to Joan Gussow, a leading nutrition educator at Columbia Teachers College, "Experimental studies as early as the turn of the century showed protein requirements to be relatively modest – quite close, in fact, to our present Recommended Dietary Allowances (RDAs). But some influential nutritionists insisted that these studies couldn't be relied upon alone."

Instead, researchers like Carl Voit, a famous German physiologist, argued that recommended protein levels ought to reflect what people actually eat. In 1881, Voit analyzed the diets of German men and, on the basis of his findings, suggested a protein intake of 118 grams each day – more than double our present RDAs. Voit's student, Wilbur Olin Atwater, became the first director of research at the United States Department of Agriculture. In the early 1900s, Atwater, following in Voit's footsteps, used the diets of American men to set *his* guideline of 125 grams of protein per day. Subsequently, both Voit and Atwater upped their recommendations even further.

In the 1950s, popular nutrition writers like Adelle Davis were still boosting protein, explaining that, "To obtain too much is . . . probably impossible; to obtain an adequate amount is to stay young for your years."[1]

A Passion for Protein. Two decades later, in the 1970s, Frances Moore Lappé's best-selling *Diet for a Small Planet* contributed to the protein mania. The book implied that protein was a scarce commodity for non-meat-eaters, even in wealthy countries like the United States. It had thousands of people painstakingly combining peanuts and sunflower seeds, or bulgur and garbanzo beans, in an effort to make sure that they met their daily protein quota.

But in the revised edition, published in 1982, Lappé offered different advice. Referring to the earlier book, she wrote, "In combatting the myth that meat is the only way to get high-quality protein, I reinforced another myth. I gave the impression that in order to get enough protein without meat, considerable care was needed in choosing foods. Actually, it is much easier than I thought."

But the myth dies hard. In recent years, food producers have placed so much emphasis on protein content that one might have supposed the nutritional equivalent of OPEC had restricted protein production. The Beef Industry Council has claimed that "Beef is a super source of complete, high-quality protein." The American Egg Board has said that "The egg is one of the best and least expensive sources of high quality protein," and Oscar Mayer & Co. has bragged that one of their wieners contains "as much protein as an egg." These "nutrition advocates" seek to obscure their products' high – and highly undesirable – content of saturated fat and cholesterol by bedazzling the consumer with protein.

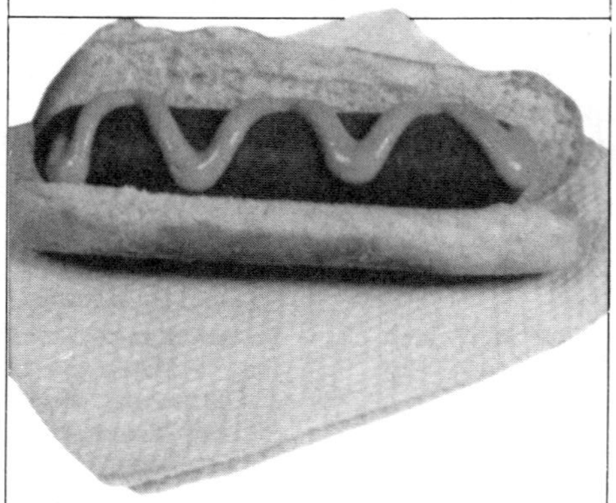

Where's The Protein? *In the hot dog and the roll – the dog has five grams, while the roll has three.*

With all this fuss, one might surmise that Americans are in dire need of protein. But according to government statistics, on average, infants and children in the United States consume about *twice* the RDA for protein. The average middle-aged man consumes 60 percent more than the recommended protein level; the average middle-aged woman about 25 percent more than recommended.[2] And less than three percent of the population gets under two-thirds of the RDA.[3] (Two-thirds is generally considered adequate, because the RDAs are constructed with generous safety margins.)

Too Much of a Good Thing? Obviously, most Americans eat plenty of protein, and some of us probably eat far too much. Among other things, excess protein may increase the risk of osteoporosis – weak, fracture-prone bones. When people eat more protein, their kidneys excrete more calcium, the mineral that keeps bones strong. If protein intake is doubled, for example, about 50 percent more calcium is lost in the urine.[4] Over time, such heavy losses could lead to osteoporosis.

Epidemiological studies of human populations also suggest a link between high-protein diets and osteoporosis. Among ten groups examined in one study, those that ate the most protein, such as Americans and New Zealanders, had the highest incidence of hip fractures, one measure of osteoporosis. Yet these groups also consumed the most calcium.[5]

People who are losing calcium because they're gorging on protein may be able to keep their bones strong by taking mega-doses of calcium. But by doing so they will load up their urine with calcium. The higher level of calcium in the urine may cause kidney stones in a small number of people.

The Old-Fashioned Kidney. One of the kidney's jobs is to rid the body of nitrogen-containing waste products from protein. But the human body evolved during the eons when humans were hunter-gatherers, and ate large, protein-rich meat meals only rarely. According to Barry Brenner of Harvard Medical School, the kidney probably needs periods of rest. So although people who live in most wealthy countries now regard a continuous high protein intake as "normal," their kidneys may not agree.

Observations of aging laboratory animals suggest that high-protein diets may damage the kidney. "If there were nursing homes for old rats, they'd be full of animals with kidney disease," says kidney researcher Mackenzie Walser of the Johns Hopkins University School of Medicine. "All laboratory rats develop this as they age."

But according to Brenner, kidney disease can be avoided by feeding the animals low-protein diets instead of protein-rich laboratory chow. Similarly, he speculates, if people reduced their protein intake, they might ward off the mild loss of kidney function that typically occurs with aging.

This age-related decline isn't important for most people. But some individuals need all the kidney function they can get. Patients with diabetes and other diseases that impair the kidney are in this category; so, too, may be people who have donated or in some other way lost a kidney. Brenner says protein restriction might help preserve vital kidney function in these individuals.

Low-protein diets (with less than three-quarters of the RDA) are known to decrease weakness, fatigue, and other symptoms in patients with failing kidneys, simply because these diets give the kidneys less work to do.[6] Relieving symptoms with a careful diet is preferable to using a dialysis machine. Furthermore, although damaged kidneys usually grow progressively worse, there's evidence, according to Walser, that low-protein diets (some as low as one-quarter or less of the RDA) can slow this relentless deterioration.

The Heart of the Matter. It's taken the American public a while to grow accustomed to the idea that diet influences heart disease. And since studies first showed this to be true, the most obvious villains – saturated fat and cholesterol – have captured most of our attention. But excess animal protein may also play a role.

According to biochemist Kenneth K. Carroll of the University of Western Ontario, "There's no doubt that, in laboratory animals, you can increase cholesterol levels by feeding large [twice the usual] amounts of casein." (Scientists often use casein, or milk protein, in experiments as a representative animal protein.) On the other hand, even huge amounts of soy protein, a widely used

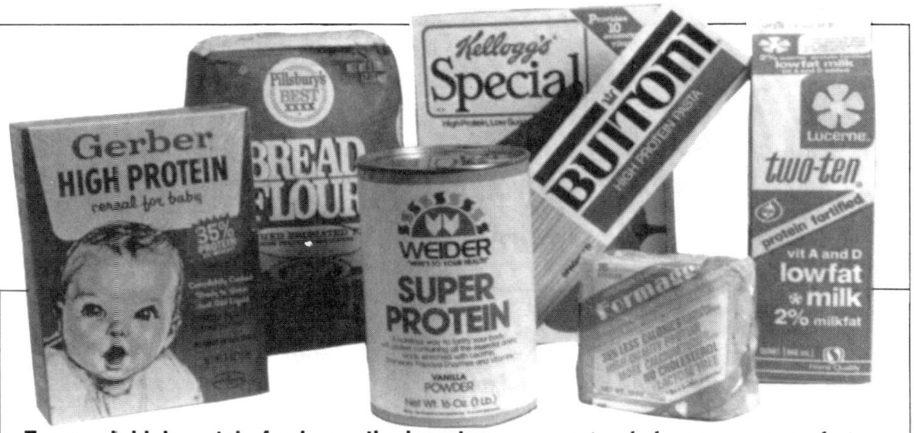

Too much high-protein food over the long term *may not only be unnecessary, but also harmful.*

plant protein, do not affect cholesterol levels.

Studies of the diets and heart disease rates of different human populations also point a warning finger at animal protein. Some of these studies found heart disease to be at least as strongly linked with animal protein in the diet as with animal fat.[7] Also, a few experiments in humans suggest that animal protein raises blood cholesterol, while vegetable protein lowers it.[8]

But some heart researchers remain skeptical. William E. Connor, of the Oregon Health Sciences University in Portland, says, "I don't think the kind or amount of protein has a decisive influence on heart disease. We don't eat protein, we eat food. And it's the company the protein keeps that has the decisive influence."

The company animal protein keeps, of course, in commonly-eaten foods such as meat, eggs, cheese, and whole milk, is saturated fat and cholesterol. And avoiding *those* troublemakers is reason enough to cut back on many animal foods while awaiting the final outcome of debates about protein.

Protein and Cancer. In a 1982 report entitled *Diet, Nutrition, and Cancer,* a committee of the National Academy of Sciences (NAS) stated, "Evidence from both epidemiological and laboratory studies suggests that high protein intake *may* be associated with an increased risk of cancers at certain sites." Specifically, the report explained, "Protein has often been associated with cancers of the breast, endometrium, [colon, rectum,] pancreas, and kidney."

As with heart disease, some studies of cancer incidence have shown as strong a link with dietary protein – especially animal protein – as with fat, but these findings have been largely ignored. "People say you can't separate out the effects of protein and the effects of fat. Then they attribute any negative effect to fat," notes Colin Campbell, a cancer researcher at Cornell University and one of the authors of the NAS report.

In animal experiments, scientists *can* separate the effects of protein from those of fat. In some of these experiments, Campbell says, animal protein promotes cancer more dramatically than does fat.

The cancer-preventing effects of reducing protein intake can be dramatic as well. In rats exposed to the carcinogen aflatoxin B, Campbell finds that animals given less protein show fewer early signs of liver cancer.[9]

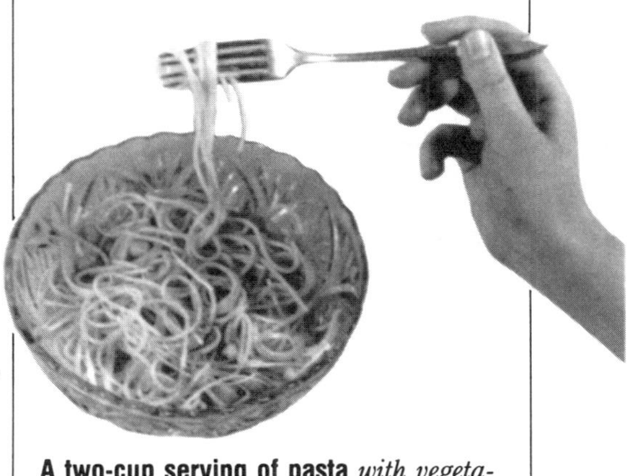

A two-cup serving of pasta *with vegetables and herbs makes a satisfying meal that contains about one-third of the USRDA for protein.*

Ervin J. Hawrylewicz, a researcher at Mercy Hospital and Medical Center in Chicago, has performed similar experiments on a strain of rats susceptible to breast cancer. After they are exposed to carcinogens, Hawrylewicz says, the animals fed diets high in casein always develop more breast tumors than those whose diets contain less casein.[10]

CONTINUED ON NEXT PAGE

W**hen you cut back on animal protein, you are apt to eat less fat and more fiber.**

CONTINUED FROM PAGE 5

Hawrylewicz also finds that high-fat diets cause tumors. But if rats on high-fat diets are fed extra casein, they develop even more tumors. Hawrylewicz concludes that protein and fat stimulate tumor growth in different ways, and that their effects can be additive.

Cutting Back is Hard to Do. Clearly, it makes sense to try to keep the protein in your diet close to the RDA. But this can be surprisingly difficult.

When CSPI staffers, for example, prepared a healthful seven-day diet (*NAH*, Jan./Feb. 1987) they tried to limit protein to 100 percent of the USRDA (USRDAs are adaptations of the RDAs that apply to everyone) while including milk, meat, and fish. It wasn't easy, because the adult USRDA for protein works out to be only about seven to ten percent of daily calories, and animal foods are typically packed with protein.

Even starchy staples, such as bread and spaghetti, get about 12 percent of their calories from protein. (Since it comes from plants, however, this protein probably has much less potential for harm than excess animal protein.) Also, when you're keeping protein intake low, it can be a challenge to consume sufficient iron and calcium—though calcium needs probably decrease when less protein is eaten.

On the positive side, when you cut back on animal protein, you are apt to eat less fat and cholesterol, and more fiber. All of these changes fit together, and all of them are steps toward better health.

Laurie Quint contributed to this article.

Footnotes

[1]Davis, A., *Let's Eat Right to Keep Fit* (New York: Harcourt, Brace and Company, 1954), p. 34.
[2]*NHANES II: 1976-1980 Consumption Data*, Series 11, No. 231.
[3]*USDA Nationwide Food Consumption Survey 1977-78: Report No. 1-2.*
[4]*Am. J. Clin. Nutr. 36:* 986, 1982.
[5]*J. Nutr. 116:* 2316, 1986.
[6]*Lancet 1:* 597, 1986.
[7]*N.Y. State J. Med. 57:* 2343, 1957.
[8]*Lancet 1:* 275, 1977.
[9]*Nutr. Cancer 3:* 200, 1982.
[10]*Nutr. Rep. Int. 26:* 793, 1982.

LESS STEAK, MORE PASTA

Here are some simple guidelines for cutting down on protein, especially animal protein.

1. Use meat and poultry as *condiments*, rather than as the centerpiece of each meal. Use small amounts to good advantage in stir-fried combination dishes, soups, stews, and casseroles.

2. Use cookbooks that feature interesting ways to prepare grains, legumes, pasta, and vegetables. *Jane Brody's Good Food Book* (Norton, 1985) and Patricia Gregory's *Bean Banquets* (Woodbridge Press, 1984) are two excellent choices.

3. Eat at least one meal a day with little or no animal protein. Try a fresh vegetable salad or stir-fry for lunch; pasta with marinara sauce for dinner.

4. Snack on high-carbohydrate, low-protein foods, such as fresh and dried fruits, raw vegetable slices, whole-grain crackers, popcorn, and juices.

5. Systematically plan a lower-protein diet, using a computer program if possible. It's tough to do this even with a computer, but it's much more difficult without.

RECOMMENDED DIETARY ALLOWANCES FOR PROTEIN

	AGE *(years)*	PROTEIN *(grams)**
Children	1-3	**23**
	4-6	**30**
	7-10	**34**
Males	11-14	**45**
	15+	**56**
Females	11-18	**46**
	19+	**44**
Pregnant		**30****
Lactating		**20****

* One ounce equals 28 grams.
** If you're pregnant, add 30 grams to the figure given for your age group; if you're breastfeeding, add 20 grams.

Source: Recommended Dietary Allowances, National Academy of Sciences-National Research Council, Revised 1980.

PROTEIN SCOREBOARD

This chart shows the protein content of commonly-eaten foods, expressed as a percent of the USRDA. Add up the values for a typical meal, and you'll see how easy it is to obtain enough protein in the course of a day. For example, a lunch consisting of a peanut butter sandwich (2 Tb. peanut butter, 2 slices whole-wheat bread) and one glass of milk provides 42 percent of the USRDA for protein. A dinner of roasted chicken (4 ounces), brown rice (1 cup), and peas (½ cup) supplies 93 percent.

FOOD	PROTEIN *(% of USRDA)**
Pork chop, trimmed, (4 oz.)	**82**
Chicken, light, w/o skin (4 oz.)	**78**
Sirloin steak, trimmed, (4 oz.)	**71**
White tuna, water pack, drained (3 oz.)	**67**
Ground beef, lean, (4 oz.)	**62**
Flounder, (4 oz.)	**51**
Cheese pizza (1 slice)	**33**
Low-fat cottage cheese (½ cup)	**31**
Lentils or split peas, cooked (1 cup)	**25**
Cheddar cheese (1½ oz.)	**24**
Milk (1 cup)	**18**
Peanut butter (2 Tb.)	**15**
Peas, cooked (1 cup)	**14**
Egg (1)	**13**
Hot dog (1)	**13**
Whole-wheat bread (2 slices)	**9**
Spaghetti, cooked (1 cup)	**9**
Brown rice, cooked (1 cup)	**8**
Corn, cooked (1 cup)	**8**
White rice, cooked (1 cup)	**6**
Post 40% Bran Flakes (⅔ cup)	**5**

* The USRDA for animal protein is 45 grams; for vegetable protein, 65 grams.

Sources: USDA Handbooks 8-1, 8-5, 8-7, 8-13, and USDA Home & Garden Bulletin 72.

Name ____________________

Section ____________________

Date ____________________

Chapter 6
QUESTIONS FOR REVIEW

1. The basic structure of a protein is an amino acid.

2. Those amino acids that the body cannot make are called essential amino acids.

3. A complete protein has all the essential amino acids in the needed amounts. Three examples of this kind of protein are:

   a. eggs

   b. milk

   c. soybeans /meats/ cheese

4. A partially complete protein has all the essential amino acids but one in the needed amounts. Two examples of this protein are:

   a. legumes (seeds)

   b. grain

5. A protein deficiency that occurs in children throughout the world is called marasmus + [kwashiorkor].

6. What is the difference between a vegan and a lacto-ovo vegetarian?

   a. vegan

   b. lacto-ovo vegetarian

7. The protein requirement is the same/different for men and women. The RDA for protein is .8 grams/kg body weight/day.

8. Most Americans consume too much/not enough dietary protein.

9. List three functions of proteins in the body.

   a. essential amino acids

   b. provide nitrogen so body make non essential

   c. protein synthesis

10. Extra protein beyond that needed is converted to ______fat______ in the body.

11. Serious weight lifters or body builders should consume a lot of extra protein per day to maximize muscle growth. (TRUE/FALSE)

CHAPTER 7

Vitamins — Water-Soluble

Probably more misinformation exists about the role of vitamins in health than all other nutrients combined. The public perception is that vitamins are healthful and that the diet is over-processed and thus deficient in vitamins. Therefore, many believe that one needs to consume vitamin supplements for proper health. Another recent trend is toward taking larger and larger doses of vitamins. What people forget is that vitamins are chemicals that have specific functions in the body. When not enough of a vitamin is present in the diet over a period of time, the metabolic process in which the vitamin normally participates no longer functions. This leads to deficiency symptoms and death in the case of some vitamin deficiencies. Different vitamins have different deficiency symptoms because each vitamin functions at different places in the metabolic pathway. Although vitamin deficiency symptoms have been described as long ago as 6,000 years, it is only since the early 1900s that the specific chemical role of vitamins has been elucidated. In fact, the biochemical role of vitamin B_{12} has only been known since 1950.

Vitamin toxicity

While the reasons for vitamin deficiency symptoms have become understood, the nutritionist now has a different problem — *vitamin toxicities.* Why is this a recent problem for nutritionists? Because until the advent and corresponding increased public use of vitamin supplements, it was impossible to consume enough excess vitamins in one's food to cause toxic symptoms. In recent years as vitamin supplementation has increased, nutritionists and physicians have discovered that vitamin toxicities have increased dramatically. Vitamins which were previously thought to be harmless have been found to cause toxicities. When overly large doses are taken, vitamins no longer work as vitamins but have drug-like actions often resulting in these toxic effects.

Vitamins are defined as *organic compounds* (complex molecules) that are *needed by the body in small amounts.* Since vitamins cannot be synthesized by the body, they need to be *consumed with the foods we eat.* Vitamins function in the body by allowing *metabolic reactions* to occur.

Fat-soluble — water-soluble vitamins

Vitamins are classified into two groups: fat-soluble and water-soluble vitamins (Table 7-1). The fat-soluble vitamins are stored in the body to a much greater degree than the water-soluble vitamins. Because fat-soluble vitamins have a *high tissue saturation* level (that is, excesses consumed in the diet are stored in body tissues), fat-soluble vitamin deficiencies take much longer to develop than water-soluble vitamin deficiencies. If a person fails to consume his requirement for a fat-soluble vitamin, it is taken from the body stores. This doesn't mean that water-soluble vitamins aren't stored, but storage is much less than that of fat-soluble vitamins. Water-soluble vitamins are said to have a *low tissue-saturation* level.

The downside of being able to store extra fat-soluble vitamins is that the fat-soluble vitamins are much more toxic than the water-soluble vitamins. Since the body accumulates fat-soluble vitamins, their effects can increase as more are stored, causing toxicities. This is especially true of vitamin D (the most toxic vitamin) and vitamin A.

When extra water-soluble vitamins are eaten, only a small amount accumulates in the body. Extra vitamins that cannot be utilized by the body are excreted in the urine. However, megadose consumption of some water-soluble vitamins has been shown to cause toxicities, as blood and tissue levels of these vitamins can increase to toxic amounts before the body can excrete the excess. Megadoses of water-soluble vitamins constantly bombard the body with *pharmacological* amounts of the vitamin. Everyone knows that two aspirin will relieve a headache, but a bottle a day over time can kill.

Table 7-1. Names of fat-soluble and water-soluble vitamins.

Fat-Soluble Vitamins	Water-Soluble Vitamins
Vitamin A	Thiamin (B_1)
Vitamin D	Riboflavin
Vitamin E	Niacin (B_2)
Vitamin K	Biotin
	Pyrodixine (B_6)
	Pantothenic Acid
	Folacin
	Vitamin B_{12}
	Ascorbic Acid (Vitamin C)

Diet variety precludes deficiencies

Vitamin deficiencies generally occur because the diet is *lacking in variety*. A limited diet means limited vitamin intake because every food does not contain every vitamin. If one does not consume a diet containing foods from the basic four food groups, his diet may lack some vitamins. Other ways in which vitamin deficiences can occur are:

1. A person's *diet totally lacks a certain vitamin.* For instance, a true vegetarian (vegan) eats a diet totally lacking in vitamin B_{12}, since this vitamin is only found in animal products. The adult vegan can develop a vitamin B_{12} deficiency after about 5 years. However, in children consuming a strict vegetarian diet, a B_{12} deficiency could occur much faster than in the adult.
2. A person *cannot absorb a vitamin.* Many intestinal diseases exist that interfere with vitamin absorption. Luckily, it is often possible to inject vitamins directly into the body, thus by-passing the problem.

3. A person has an *increased requirement for a vitamin.* Recent research has shown that during growth a person's need for certain vitamins increases. Other research shows that the use of estrogen birth control pills, excessive amounts of alcohol, intakes of excessive amounts of dietary protein and excessive expenditures of energy (as in intensive aerobic training), all increase one's requirement for certain vitamins. Most of the time these factors cause only a small increase (perhaps 10%) above a person's normal requirement. Contrary to the food faddist's claims, one does not need megadose intakes to ovecome these problems.

Co-enzymes

Water-soluble vitamins generally function as *co-enzymes* in the body (Table 7-1). A co-enzyme is a chemical that is necessary before an enzyme can work. All of the metabolic processes in the body are really a series of short reactions that are controlled by enzymes. For example, to convert glucose to energy at least 50 different metabolic steps are required. Each of these metabolic steps requires an enzyme, and vitamins function as co-enzymes in many of these steps. The absence of a vitamin will prevent a reaction from occurring because the enzyme can no longer function without its co-enzyme. But it is very important to understand that an excess of a vitamin *cannot* increase or speed up reactions.

If a vitamin is necessary for the production of muscle, a deficiency of that vitamin will slow muscle synthesis. But an excess of that vitamin *will not* cause one to produce extra muscles. An everyday analogy is that a car needs four tires to function properly. It will not run very well on one or two tires and may not run at all if it has no tires. But having fifteen or fifty tires available does not make the car run any better because it can only use four at a time. When one understands that vitamins do not directly control metabolic reactions but only allow biochemical reactions to proceed, one can more easily understand that large excesses of vitamins are mostly ineffective and cannot work as some people (often people trying to sell you vitamins) suggest. Excessive intakes of some vitamins can affect various metabolic processes in the body (such as high intakes of niacin to reduce blood cholesterol levels). These effects are pharmacological (drug-like) and not related to the vitamin function.

Water-Soluble Vitamins

In this course, you need to only be aware of some general functions of a few of the vitamins. These vitamins include niacin, pyridoxine, vitamin B_{12} and ascorbic acid.

Niacin

Niacin: As with all of the vitamins, niacin has an interesting history, especially in the United States. A deficiency of niacin is called pellegra, meaning rough skin. In the early 1900s in the United States, pellegra accounted for as many as 10,000 deaths per year. Pellegra occurred primarily in the South and eventually was attributed to the diet that was eaten by poor southerners.

Pellegra is characterized by the four D's: *dermatitis* (rough skin), *diarrhea, dementia* (mental problems) and *death.* Niacin as a vitamin acts as co-enzyme in many metabolic reactions throughout the body. Problems are first noticed in the skin and intestine, because these tissues are more metabolically active and are therefore the first to be affected by a deficiency. Also, it is easy to see changes in the skin or notice changes in bowel movements as compared to changes in the kidneys. As the deficiency continues, a lack of niacin affects brain hormones, leading to mental imbalance. Eventually, the niacin deficiency affects so many systems in the body that death occurs. Figure 7-1 illustrates the typical dermatitis of pellegra.

As previously mentioned, the foods eaten by poor, rural southerners contained little niacin. Their diet consisted primarily of the three "M" foods: *milk, molasses* and *maize* (corn). The continual consumption of these foods with very little fresh fruits, vegetables, or whole grains eventually produced pellegra.

Figure 7-1. An example of the dermatitis associated with pellegra. (From Pyke, M. *Man & Foods*, McGraw Hill Book Co., 1970.)

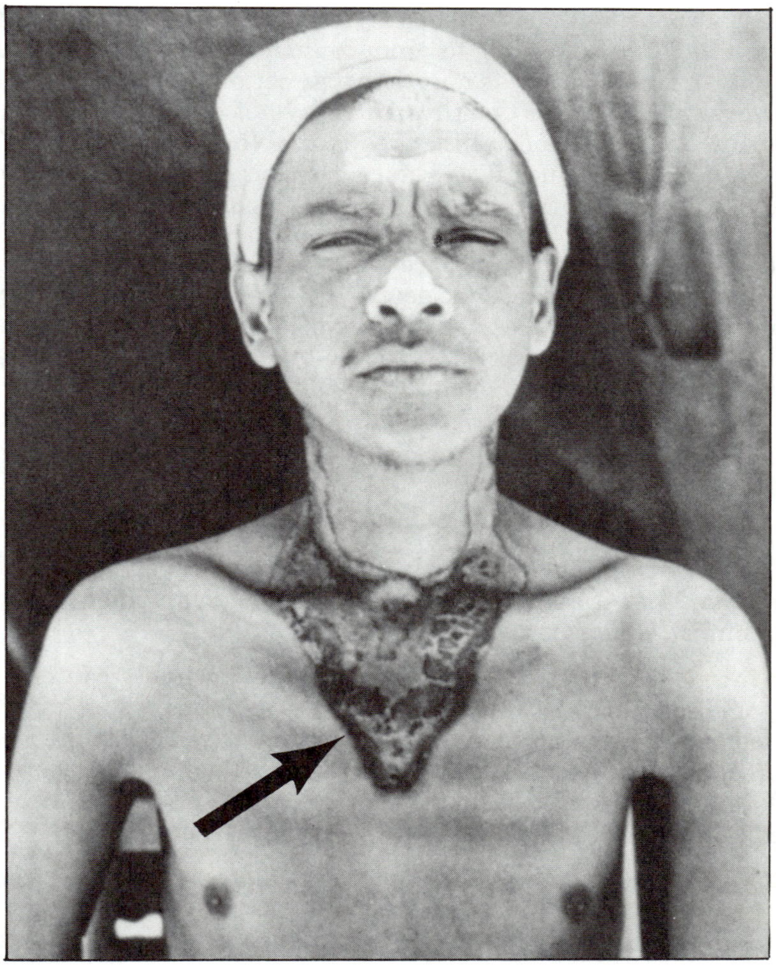

Pyridoxine: The vitamin pyridoxine is included for discussion in this chapter because it has become increasingly popular as a nutritional supplement. Large doses of pyridoxine have been suggested as therapeutic or beneficial in relieving the symptoms of premenstrual syndrome (PMS), jet lag, and numbness of the hands and fingers (carpal tunnel syndrome). Unfortunately, controlled experiments have failed to find these treatments effective. As so often occurs, it is the placebo effect that seems to cause the beneficial responses to this vitamin.

Pyridoxine

Pyridoxine's main function is as a *co-enzyme in reactions affecting protein and amino acid metabolism.* A deficiency of pyridoxine can negatively affect protein synthesis in the body. As a result, megadose supplements have become increasingly popular in athletes, especially weightlifters and body builders. The rationale is that if pyridoxine is needed for protein metabolism, intakes of megadoses of pyridoxine will stimulate protein synthesis. *WRONG!* Again, a co-enzyme cannot stimulate a metabolic reaction above what normally would occur. It is true that excessive protein intake, such as some weightlifters consume, does cause a slightly increased need for pyridoxine because pyridoxine is necessary to metabolize this extra protein. However, the increase is small compared with the megadose intakes some athletes are consuming.

The RDA for pyridoxine is 2 mg/day. Even when consuming large amounts of extra protein, a person's pyridoxine need would never be more than 3 mg/day — a 50% increase. The suggested therapeutic doses of pyridoxine to relieve pre-menstrual syndrome is 500 mg/day or 250 times the RDA. Weightlifters have been known to consume 5000 mg/day or more supposedly to maximize protein (muscle) accumulation. This amount is 2500 times the requirement. If this extra intake were just costing a person money, then most nutritionists, while not endorsing the procedure, would not be as opposed. However, in the last few years cases have been reported of pyridoxine toxicity. Persons consuming 5000 mg of pyridoxine per day for one to two months started complaining of numbness in the arms and legs, loss of muscular function and even paralysis. Although these cases are rare, in all instances when the person stopped consuming the pyridoxine the symptoms gradually disappeared. As we have learned more about pyridoxine toxicity, it appears that long-term (2-3 years) consumption of moderate intakes of pyridoxine (200-500 mg/day) also causes the same toxicity symptoms.

Vitamin B_{12}: Only since the 1950s have nutritionists known that this vitamin was required for humans. A deficiency of vitamin B_{12} is called *pernicious anemia*. Many years ago a person who developed the symptoms associated with pernicious anemia always died (although at the time it was not known what caused this death). Pernicious anemia is characterized in the early stages by anemia (decreased number of red blood cells in the blood). In the latter stages nerve degeneration occurs, leading to paralysis and eventually death. Vitamin B_{12} has two major functions in the body: *red blood cell production* and *nerve tissue production.*

B_{12}

Vitamin B_{12} deficiency is unique in that it can occur even though a person's diet contains normal amounts of vitamin B_{12}. In the 1920s it was discovered that in order to absorb vitamin B_{12} into the body the vitamin needs to be attached to a protein. This protein, made in the stomach, is called intrinsic factor. People that were unable to make the intrinsic factor protein could not absorb vitamin B_{12}, and they invariably died of pernicious anemia.

Vitamin B_{12} is only found in *animal products* with the best source being *liver*. Starting in the late 1920s it was discovered that if people with the inability to produce intrinsic factor ate ½ to 1 pound of *raw* liver per day, they would consume enough vitamin B_{12} so that even without intrinsic factor, enough vitamin B_{12} would be absorbed to keep their nerves from degenerating. While this may not seem very palatable, most people readily adapted to the raw liver diet. Cooking, unfortunately, destroys most of the vitamin B_{12}.

Eventually vitamin B_{12} was purified and synthesized in the laboratory. Now persons with an inability to absorb vitamin B_{12} can receive a B_{12} shot, by-passing the metabolic problem. Other groups often receive vitamin B_{12} shots. The elderly, as they age, stop producing intrinsic factor. Thus, it is standard practice in geriatric medicine to give the elderly a B_{12} shot every 6 months. Also, one often hears of athletes getting B_{12} shots when they are tired or ill with a cold. This is totally unnecessary except as a placebo treatment unless the athlete cannot make intrinsic factor (very rare).

Another group that has to be somewhat concerned about its vitamin B_{12} status is true vegetarians (vegans). Since vitamin B_{12} is only found in animal products, adult vegans could develop vitamin B_{12} deficiency after about 4-5 years of meatless eating. We require very little vitamin B_{12} as illustrated by the years it takes to develop a deficiency. If a vegan eats animal products as little as once or twice a year, he will receive enough vitamin B_{12} for another year.

Ascorbic acid

Ascorbic Acid: This vitamin, also commonly known as vitamin C, is a water-soluble vitamin about which nutrition misinformation abounds. Ascorbic acid is only a vitamin for man, primates, guinea pigs and a few exotic species. The rest of the animal kingdom is able to make as much ascorbic acid as needed without added dietary intake. Ascorbic acid deficiency symptoms in humans, called *scurvy*, have been recognized for as long as 3000 years although it wasn't known what caused the symptoms.

In isolated villages in Europe during the Middle Ages, scurvy would often occur as the winter lengthened and fresh foods were no longer available. However, it was during the long sea voyages of the 1500s and 1600s that scurvy became most widespread and recognized as a serious problem. On some long voyages as many as 90-95% of the sailors would develop scurvy. Eventually crude experiments were conducted in which different groups of sailors were given different rations during the voyages. It was discovered that those sailors receiving limes were the least susceptible to scurvy. This ration was introduced as standard fare by the British Navy and the sailors became known as "limeys."

Figure 7-3. Examples of Scurvy: Panel A shows gum degeneration; Panel B shows pinpoint bleeding. (From Pyke, M. *Man & Food)* McGraw-Hill Book Co., 1970)

Understanding the main functions of ascorbic acid allows one to understand how the deficiency symptoms of scurvy develop. The main function of ascorbic acid is in the production of *collagen*. Collagen is the "glue" that holds the cells together. Many of the signs of scurvy result from the body's inability to produce collagen. Other functions of ascorbic acid are:

1. to function in bone metabolism,
2. to aid in the production of brain hormones,
3. to aid in the production of immune factors.

The deficiency symptoms of scurvy are listed in Table 7-2.

Because ascorbic acid deficiency causes a reduction in immune function, some people, most notably Linus Pauling, have suggested that extra ascorbic acid can prevent or reduce the severity of colds. The rationale is that the extra ascorbic acid will boost the immune system's function, thereby protecting one from catching a cold. The RDA for ascorbic acid is *60 mg per day*. This is about the amount found in 1 small orange. Food faddists suggest that one needs to consume megadoses of ascorbic acid (from 1,000 to 10,000 mg per day) to prevent colds.

Is there any evidence that taking large doses of ascorbic acid will lessen your chances of catching a cold? Most *controlled, double-blind* experiments have failed to find any benefit from consuming large doses of ascorbic acid. The experiments need to be double-blind because it is very important that neither the subject nor the investigator know whether the subject is receiving the ascorbic acid supplement or a control. This eliminates any placebo effect of the treatment and allows valid conclusions to be drawn. Be very leery of any nutritional claims that rely on personal testimony. Unfortunately, even if one took ascorbic acid supplements and said he had fewer colds during the previous year because of them, as scientists we would still conclude that this was because of the placebo effect, not an actual effect of the ascorbic acid. The studies must be controlled and double-blind for them to mean anything scientifically.

Table 7-2. Scurvy deficiency symptoms in order of development.

Deficiency Symptoms	Reason
1. pinpoint bleeding on the surface of the body	lack of collagen allows cells to pull apart — causes capillaries to burst
2. bleeding gums	lack of collagen allows free bleeding
3. sore joints and bones	ascorbic acid's function in bone metabolism impaired
4. mental disorders	brain hormone balance changed
5. scars open up	lack of collagen
6. increased infections	decreased production of antibodies
7. death	usually due to increased infections

From the many controlled studies that have taken place in the last 15 years and because many people take megadose amounts of ascorbic acid, nutritionists have been able to document ascorbic acid toxicities. While these toxicities are variable, not occurring to the same extent in every person receiving the same dose of ascorbic acid, they occur often enough to be considered serious.

Table 7-3 lists some of the toxic side effects of excessive ascorbic acid consumption. These toxicities are real. The more ascorbic acid one consumes, the more likely he is to experience toxic side effects. Ascorbic acid is a potent chemical of the class known as reducers. If you are going to take an ascorbic acid supplement, take 500 mg or less per day. Although nutritionists are discovering more each day about ascorbic acid toxicities (because the longer people consume them, the more we learn about the toxic effects), it appears that the effects of 500 mg per day are much less severe than with larger supplement intakes. If you are convinced that only ascorbic acid supplements will protect you from getting the flu, limit your intake to 500 mg or less per day.

Table 7-3. Toxicity associated with excessive ascorbic acid intakes.

1. diarrhea, bloating, cramps
2. increased incidence of kidney stones
3. anemia — due to increased destruction of red blood cells (occurs in black and Asian populations primarily)
4. rebound scurvy (scurvy-like symptoms occur after one stops taking large doses of ascorbic acid)
5. infantile scurvy (scurvy-like symptoms can develop in infants born to mothers taking large doses of ascorbic acid while pregnant)

The vitamin pushers

From drug company to drug store, sellers tell you that you need vitamin supplements. Do you really?

The more things change, the more they remain the same. When CU was founded 50 years ago, we published a report, called "The Vitamin Stampede," that deplored the overselling of vitamins to the U.S. population.

Dr. Walter C. Alvarez of the Mayo Clinic, the author of our 1936 report, said that vitamins were being "forced on children and adults without sufficient thought and understanding."

At that time, some experiments had suggested that a certain vitamin might help to prevent colds. But more-careful, controlled trials had indicated, as Dr. Alvarez put it, "that these substances cannot be counted on to influence respiratory infections." Vitamin C? No, it was vitamin A back then.

Today, the buzz words for selling vitamins have been modernized—even though vitamins themselves, and the human body's limited need for them, have remained the same. A recent trend is to push vitamins for the relief of "stress." Almost everyone, of course, experiences stress. If it follows that nearly everyone needs vitamins pills, commercial logic is satisfied even if science is not.

As part of our research for this report, we sent reporters, posing as customers, to 30 pharmacies in Pennsylvania, Missouri, and California (see box opposite). Our customers told the pharmacist that they'd been feeling nervous or tired lately, and asked whether a vitamin would help. Neither nervousness nor tiredness calls for vitamin supplementation. But most of the 30 pharmacists seemed more than willing to sell vitamin pills for those purposes. And only nine mentioned the possibility of seeing a doctor. Ethics put in the pocket? Or just inadequate professional knowledge? Either way, we had hoped for better.

Pharmacists are only one part of the picture. Drug-company advertising is another big part. Pushed by the ads, the public has developed quite an appetite for vitamin pills. Sales of vitamins in the U.S. are close to $3-billion a year. Surveys suggest that about half of all Americans pop a vitamin pill either regularly or occasionally—and some people take a handful or more every day.

Most vitamin users, concerned that their diet may not be adequate, take their daily doses as "insurance" against deficiency. Others—operating on the mistaken theory that if some is good, more must be better—hope that the products will provide extra energy, prevent disease, protect against stress, or enhance athletic ability.

What vitamins are

A vitamin is an organic substance required to promote one or more essential biochemical reactions within living cells. Unlike foods, vitamins are needed only in tiny amounts and are not a source of energy (calories).

For a substance to qualify as a vitamin, its absence must cause a specific deficiency disease that is cured when the substance is resupplied. (Lack of vitamin C, for example, causes scurvy.) It may take weeks or months for any signs of deficiency to show up.

There are 13 known vitamins required by humans. Four are fat-soluble (A, D, E, and K), and nine are water-soluble (C and the eight "B-complex" vitamins—thiamin, riboflavin, niacin, B_6, folic acid, B_{12}, pantothenic acid, and biotin). Do any more remain to be discovered? Probably not, since patients have survived for years on intravenous feedings fortified with only these vitamins. Non-vitamins such as P, B_{15}, and B_{17} continue to be touted by hucksters as vitamins, but they are not and never have been.

How much you need

The Food and Nutrition Board of the National Research Council/National Academy of Sciences publishes guidelines known as the Recommended Dietary Allowances (RDAs). These are defined as "the levels of intake of essential nutrients considered adequate to meet the known nutritional needs of practically all healthy persons."

The RDAs are not "minimums" or "requirements." The level for each nutrient is deliberately set higher than most people need. The RDA for each vitamin is usually derived by estimating the range of normal human needs, selecting the number at the high end of that range, and adding a safety factor. The values vary somewhat by age and sex, and are increased for women during pregnancy and breast-feeding.

For three vitamins—K, pantothenic acid, and biotin—the Food and Nutrition Board has published "estimated safe and adequate intakes" rather than RDAs. This was done because part of people's need for those vitamins is supplied by bacteria within the intestines; how much must come from food is not known.

The U.S. Food and Drug Administration took the National Research Council's figures and simplified them to create the U.S. Recommended Daily Allowances (U.S. RDAs), which you see on many food labels. U.S. RDAs generally represent the highest level of the NRC's Recommended Dietary Allowance for each nutrient. Therefore, few if any people need more

This article is reprinted courtesy of *Consumer Report*, March 1986, pp. 170-175.

than the U.S. RDA. Most people can do just fine on less.

Crying wolf

Many vitamin advocates suggest that everyone should take supplements to be sure that they get enough. They say, for example, that "eating on the run" and "overprocessing" of foods place the typical American in danger of deficiency.

Some also speak of "soil depletion" and dieting as reasons why people need vitamin supplements. CU's medical consultants believe that such arguments amount to crying wolf.

It's true that eating on the run, skipping entire meals, and watching one's weight have become common for many Americans. But it's unlikely that those habits are breeding vitamin deficiencies.

Take fast foods, for starters. When we last looked at Wendy's, Pizza Hut, McDonald's and their cohorts (CONSUMER REPORTS, July 1984), we commented that fast-food meals can be reasonably nutritious, especially if you use the salad bar. The main problem with fast food is not what's missing but what's there—a lot of calories, sodium, and fat.

Skipping meals? Certainly, many people do it. But people who eat only one or two meals daily during the week usually more than make up for any deficits with snacks and with increased variety and abundance on weekends.

Dieting should be done sensibly, of course. But only prolonged or highly unbalanced diets could create any risk of vitamin deficiency, CU's medical consultants say.

The argument about "overprocessing" of foods oversimplifies a complex issue. Processing can remove some vitamins and other nutrients. But it can also restore them or add new ones.

Our consultants scoff at the idea that depleted soil robs the American diet of vitamins. A plant's mineral content may be influenced by soil composition, but its vitamin content is largely determined by the plant's heredity.

Finally, some vitamins are lost in cooking. But losses of that sort are usually only partial, and are taken into account in the recommendation to include uncooked fruits and vegetables in your diet.

'Nutrition insurance'

The suggestion to buy "nutrition insurance" in pill form can be very appealing. A flyer from General Nutrition Corp., which operates almost 1300 health-food stores, states the case simply: "It would take a computer and a good deal of conscious effort to devise a diet that each day would give all the nutrients in optimum amounts . . . From the viewpoint of . . . nutrition, a complete supplement may be the best possible buy in health insurance."

But experts disagree. "Vitamin pushers use deception by omission," states Victor Herbert, Professor of Medicine at Mount Sinai School of Medicine in New York City. "They list all the terrible things that can happen if your diet is lacking. But they never tell you that vitamin deficiency is rare unless a person's diet is extremely unbalanced. Most important, they never tell how to measure whether or not your diet is adequate. If they did, they'd lose customers. Determining dietary adequacy is actually quite easy."

Easy and undramatic. You can get an adequate amount of all essential nutrients by planning your meals to include what nutritionists call the Basic Four Food Groups. Your average daily intake should include:

- Four servings of vegetables, fruits and fruit juices, at least one of which should be fresh.
- Four servings of grain and cereal products (including cereals, breads, rice, macaroni, and the like).
- Two to four servings of meats or alternatives such as fish, poultry, eggs, or beans.
- Two to four servings of milk or dairy products.

Because foods within each group differ in nutrient content, choosing a variety within each group is important. Adhering to the recommended minimum, with reasonable portion sizes, would provide about 1200 calories and adequate amounts of all essential nutrients. Since most people eat more than that, it should be clear that eating a wide variety of foods from the Basic Four will easily provide the nutrients you need. Further, though some advocates would lead you to believe otherwise, a few days without one vitamin or another will do you no real harm.

Hype about stress

If the "nutrition-insurance" appeal is old hat, the new ploy in selling vitamins is to offer you protection against "stress." While some vitamin promoters refer only to physical stresses, others include mental stress, overwork, and the like. And some make no health claims at all, but rely on the word "stress" in the product's name to sell it.

Typical "stress-formula" vitamin products contain 10 or more times the RDA for vitamin C and for several of the B-vitamins.

The Sears Shop at Home Service, which markets ***Puritan's Pride*** stress formulas, asserts that "active lives subject us to considerable stress. Working hard and even playing hard create one type of stress. The weather even affects us. Colds and illness make more demands on our bodies. Of course the everyday pressures of life bring on emotional stress. All these types of stress increase your body's needs for vitamins."

The I. Magnin department store chain recommends ***Clientele Stress Control Nutrients*** "if you're very active, deal frequently with decision-making or just find yourself drained from everyday events."

A flyer from General Nutrition Corp. includes "traffic jams, arguments, meeting fast-approaching deadlines, or simply trying to decide what to wear at a party" as sources of emotional stress that "can take their toll on various nutrients in our body, especially vitamin C and B-complex vitamins."

Hoffmann-La Roche, which wholesales most of the vitamin ingredients used by other manufacturers, has advertised that "if you drink, smoke, diet or happen to be sick, you may be robbing your body of vitamins."

Where the shortages are

Although vitamin deficiences are rare among people who eat a reasonably varied diet, a fair number of Americans may need more of certain minerals. Here are three that some people—especially women—should pay special attention to.

Fluoride intake throughout childhood helps build decay-resistant teeth. The most efficient, economical way to get it is through fluoridated water. Children who grow up in nonfluoridated communities should take supplementary fluoride (by prescription) from birth through age 12.

Calcium deserves particular attention because inadequate calcium intake is a factor in the development of osteoporosis, or thinning of the bones, especially in women. Those who like milk, cheese, and other dairy products may get what they need from diet alone. But those consuming little calcium-rich food should seek advice on supplementation from a doctor or registered dietitian. (For more on this subject, see our October 1984 report on osteoporosis.)

Iron is needed to make hemoglobin, the component in red blood cells that carries oxygen to the tissues. Lack of sufficient iron causes iron-deficiency anemia. Women who are pregnant or who menstruate heavily should be checked by a doctor to be sure they are not anemic.

The vitamin lineup

Vitamin	U.S. RDA [1]	Functions	Sources
A (retinol)	5000 IU [2]	Helps maintain eyes, skin, linings of the nose, mouth, digestive and urinary tracts	Liver, whole milk, butter, cheese, fortified margarine, carrots, spinach, other vegetables
Thiamin (B_1)	1.5 milligrams	Helps convert carbohydrates into energy	Yeast, rice, whole-grain and enriched breads and cereals, liver, pork, lean meats, poultry, eggs, meats, fish, many fruits and vegetables
Riboflavin (B_2)	1.7 milligrams	Helps energy release; helps maintain skin, mucous membranes, and nervous structures	Dairy products, liver, yeast, fruits, whole-grain and enriched breads and cereals, vegetables, lean meats, poultry
Niacin (B_3)	20 milligrams	Helps convert carbohydrates, fats, and protein into energy; essential for growth; aids synthesis of hormones	Liver, chicken, turkey, halibut, tuna, milk, eggs, grains, fruits and vegetables, enriched breads and cereals
B_6 (pyridoxine, pyridoxal, pyridoxamine)	2.0 milligrams	Aids in more than 60 enzyme reactions	Milk, liver, lean meats, whole-grain or enriched breads and cereals, vegetables
Folic acid	0.4 milligram	Aids blood-cell production; helps maintain nervous system	Liver, many vegetables
Biotin	0.3 milligram	Aids in intermediary metabolism of fats, carbohydrates, and protein	Widely distributed in foods
Pantothenic acid	10 milligrams	Aids in metabolism of carbohydrates, fats, and protein	Eggs, liver, kidneys, peanuts, whole grains, most vegetables, fish
B_{12}	6.0 micrograms	Helps synthesis of red and white blood cells; aids many other metabolic reactions	Liver, meat, eggs, milk
C (ascorbic acid)	60 milligrams	Helps maintain and repair connective tissue, bones, teeth, cartilage; promotes wound-healing	Broccoli, brussels sprouts, citrus fruits, tomatoes, potatoes, peppers, cabbage, other fruits and vegetables
D (cholecalciferol)	400 IU [2]	Helps regulate calcium and phosphorus metabolism; promotes calcium absorption; essential for development and maintenance of bones and teeth	Fortified milk, fish-liver oils; sunlight on skin produces vitamin D
E (tocopherol)	30 IU [2]	Protects and maintains cellular membranes; protects fats and vitamin A from destruction by oxidation	Vegetable oils, whole grains, leafy vegetables; smaller amounts widespread in foods
K	70 to 140 micrograms [3]	Used in synthesis of prothrombin (essential for blood clotting)	Green leafy vegetables, soybeans, beef liver; widespread in other foods

[1] *U.S. RDA for adults and children 4 or more years of age.* [3] *Estimated safe and adequate intake.*
[2] *International Units.*

Ayerst Laboratories, stating that "just being alive is stressful," has suggested *Beminal Stress Plus* to avoid "stress burnout," a vitamin-deficiency state to which "nobody is immune."

Lederle Laboratories—makers of *Stresstabs*—has been warning for years that "stress can deplete your body's stores of water-soluble vitamins" and that "daily replacement is necessary."

According to Lederle, the market leader, the concept of high-dosage stress vitamins is based on a 1952 National Research Council report that recommended extra vitamins for people suffering from stresses such as general surgery, serious burns, and major fractures. However, the report explicity stated that "in minor illnesses or injury where the expected duration of the disease is less than 10 days and when the patient is essentially ambulatory and is eating his diet . . . a good diet will supply the recommended dietary allowances of all nutrients."

Nutrition experts advise that although vitamin needs may rise with certain physical conditions, they seldom rise above the Recommended Dietary Allowances—and are easily met by proper eating. Someone who is under enough stress to incur vitamin deficiency would probably be sick enough to be in a hospital. But ads for stress vitamins have generally been aimed at well-nourished members of the general public.

No evidence exists that *emotional* stress increases the body's need for vitamins. Leon Ellenbogen, Lederle's chief of nutritional science, states emphatically that his company does not recommend *Stresstabs* for psychological stress. "We make it clear in our ads that we're talking about physical stress."

To be sure, ads for *Stresstabs* make no mention of emotional stress. But ads like the one above do picture an executive working at a desk after dark and tout the product "for people who burn the candle at both ends"—a phrase that many people would probably interpret as emotional rather than physical stress.

"Really, we have tried very hard to communicate accurately in our advertising," Ellenbogen says. "Our product was intended to replenish supplies of water-soluble vitamins in people who for one reason or another failed to get enough in their diet. People who eat a balanced diet do not need stress vitamins—or for that matter any vitamin supplement at all. Remember, though, the risk of supplementing with RDA amounts of vitamins and minerals is nil. The real vitamin quackery is done by health-food people who suggest high-dosage supplements for just about every known ailment."

New York Attorney General Robert Abrams is trying to regulate stress-vitamin marketing. In December, E.R. Squibb & Sons, which has been marketing *Theragran Stress Formula* since mid-1984, entered an agreement with the state to modify the claims made on its packaging. Squibb had been claiming that *Theragran Stress Formula* helps relieve stress resulting from "the complications of everyday life."

Abrams had charged that Squibb had falsely represented "that taking the recommended daily allowance would reduce the effects of psychological stress." He also charged that the company had implied that biotin is difficult to obtain in an average diet, when in fact "biotin deficiency is virtually nonexistent." (Except in infants, biotin deficiency has been reported only in individuals who ate unbalanced diets containing large amounts of raw eggs, which block biotin absorption.)

Squibb paid New York State $15,000 in costs and entered the agreement without admitting wrongdoing. Abrams says that other companies are under investigation for similar claims.

Hype for athletes

Athletes, from the professional to the weekend jogger, may be tempted to pop vitamin pills to achieve better performance or to replenish vitamins lost through vigorous activity.

A cascade of advertising hypes vitamins for athletes. Revco's *Competition Plus*—"for extra effort sports"—is claimed to "meet the special nutritional needs of sports active people." *All American Sports Vitamins* are said to contain vitamins and other substances "to help you get the absolute maximum out of every ounce of sweat, every hour of training." Twinsport's *Endurance* products—endorsed by Robert Haas, author of "Eat to Win"—are claimed to help realize your potential "whether you're a world-class athlete or a weekend recreationalist." Solgar says its *Joggers* tablets are formulated "to give an edge to the serious competitor and endurance athlete." And Ayerst suggests that even a two-mile jog is reason to replenish vitamins and minerals with *Beminal Stress Plus.*

It is true that strenuous exercise increases the need for calories, water, and a few nutrients. However, vitamin needs are unlikely to rise above the RDA amounts available from a balanced diet.

The notion that extra vitamins are useful to athletes is also tied to the idea that extra vitamins provide extra energy—which is untrue. Energy comes from the calories in food, and vitamins have no caloric value. A few companies—even more fanciful—have marketed vitamins supposedly formulated for specific sports.

Hype for smokers

Smokers are known to have lower blood levels of vitamin C than do nonsmokers, which has led some promoters to suggest that smokers should take extra vitamin C. But according to Victor Herbert, "There is no credible evidence that smokers need more than RDA amounts of vitamin C. The 1980 RDA amounts are at least four times as much as a normal person would ever need in a day."

Alfred E. Harper, Professor of Biochemistry and Nutrition Sciences at the University of Wisconsin, who chaired the 1974 National Research Council RDA Committee, says, "Since most subjects used in the major experiments that served as the basis for present vitamin C allowances were smokers, the suggestion that smokers need high doses of vitamin C seems incongruous. If anything, it would seem much more appropriate to suggest that nonsmokers need less."

Dangers of excess vitamins

Fat-soluble vitamins are not excreted efficiently. They are generally stored until they can be used up, and thus can accumulate to toxic levels. For example, prolonged excessive intake of vitamin A can cause headache, increased pressure on the brain, bone pain, and damage to the liver. Excessive vitamin D can cause kidney damage.

Though the water-soluble vitamins are generally excreted quickly when taken in excess, some of them can cause trouble. Large doses of niacin can cause liver damage, severe flushes, and skin rash. High doses of vitamin C can cause diarrhea.

Some vitamin myths

Some of the claims for the health effects of various vitamins recall a wag's comment about second marriages—"a triumph of hope over experience."

Vitamin C and colds

Proponents—most notably the chemist and Nobel laureate Linus Pauling—claim that vitamin C in daily dosages of 1000 milligrams or more can help prevent colds. But at least 16 double-blind studies over the past decade have found no such benefit.

The classic study was conducted by researchers at the University of Toronto. They divided 3500 volunteers into eight groups. Two groups received 250 milligrams a day of vitamin C. Two groups received 1000 milligrams, and two received 2000 milligrams. The final two groups received a placebo.

The study concluded that vitamin C did not prevent colds at all, but might help to slightly reduce the severity of cold symptoms. To achieve this mild benefit, a daily dose of 250 milligrams (about the amount in two eight-ounce glasses of orange juice) was enough. Higher doses provided no extra benefit.

Vitamin C and cancer

Pauling also believes that massive doses of vitamin C can prolong the life of cancer patients. This claim is based on a study he reported with Ewan Cameron, a Scottish physician. However, experts who analyzed the report concluded that the study was not properly designed.

The Mayo Clinic has conducted two clinical trials to test the effectiveness of vitamin C against cancer, each involving 100 or more patients in the advanced stage of the disease. Half the patients received vitamin C, half a placebo. The researchers found no differences in survival time, appetite, severity of pain, weight loss, or amount of nausea and vomiting.

Vitamin E and breast lumps

Several years ago, preliminary studies by Dr. Robert London and colleagues at Sinai Hospital of Baltimore suggested that vitamin E supplements might help women with mammary dysplasia (also called benign fibrocystic disease of the breast). But two double-blind studies reported last year found no significant benefit. In one, the Sinai Hospital team treated 128 patients for two months with either a placebo or with 150, 300, or 600 International Units of vitamin E. Although slightly more than half the patients improved during the trial period, those receiving vitamin E did no better than those receiving the placebo. The other study, by doctors at the University of California in San Francisco, involved 62 women who took either 600 IU of vitamin E or a placebo for two months. No differences in breast findings were observed between the two groups.

B_6 for premenstrual syndrome

High dosages of vitamin B_6 have been widely advocated as a treatment for premenstrual syndrome. The evidence supporting this practice is thin—mixed results in small-scale studies. Since water-soluble vitamins are relatively safe in large doses (compared with fat-soluble vitamins), some doctors felt comfortable in recommending B_6 in the range of 200 to 800 milligrams daily. (That dose is 100 to 400 times the RDA.) Recently, however, doctors have reported seeing damage to the nervous system in individuals who took daily doses of 2000 milligrams or more of vitamin B_6 for long periods of time. Adverse effects have also shown up in a few individuals who took 500-milligram doses, and in one person whose reported intake was 200 milligrams a day for three years. Their symptoms, which resembled those of multiple sclerosis, included numbness and tingling of the hands, difficulty in walking, and electric shocks shooting down the spine.

In light of these cases, CU's medical consultants advise against megadoses of vitamin B_6.

And high doses of vitamin B_6 over long periods can cause permanent damage to the nervous system.

Reported cases of vitamin toxicity are uncommon. But they are particularly sad because most people who get into trouble with vitamins have essentially poisoned themselves in the pursuit of health.

Recommendations

CU's medical consultants believe that the best way to get vitamins is from foods in a balanced diet. Vitamin supplementation may be appropriate for children up to two years old, for children who have poor eating habits, for some people on prolonged weight-reduction programs, for pregnant women, for strict vegetarians (those who avoid eggs and milk as well as meat), and for people with certain illnesses, as directed by a physician.

Rather than taking vitamins for "insurance," evaluate your diet to determine whether you are eating a variety of foods from the Basic Four groups. If you have trouble figuring that out by yourself, record what you eat for a week and ask a registered dietitian or a physician whether you are missing anything. If you are, the best course of action will probably be to improve your eating habits.

As a rule, don't take more than the RDA amounts except on medical advice. And avoid doctors or nutrition consultants who recommend vitamins as cure-alls.

Several things can be done to clean up the vitamin marketplace:

- The Food and Drug Administration should evaluate the claims made by promoters of "stress vitamins" and publicize its findings. The FDA should also work with the pharmaceutical industry to develop voluntary standards for vitamin-product formulations.
- The Federal Trade Commission should attempt to stop misleading advertising for "nutrition insurance," "stress tablets," "sports vitamins," and the like.
- The pharmaceutical profession should recognize the pushing of unnecessary supplements as an ethical issue that deserves its serious attention.

Name ________________________

Section ________________________

Date ________________________

Chapter 7

QUESTIONS FOR REVIEW

1. Define the term vitamin.

2. Fat-soluble vitamins have high/low tissue saturation levels and are generally considered more/less toxic than water-soluble vitamins.

3. Vitamin deficiencies generally occur because a person's diet is lacking in variety. List three other reasons a person could have a vitamin deficiency.

   a.

   b.

   c.

4. Water-soluble vitamins function as ____________-____________ , allowing enzymes to work.

5. A deficiency of niacin is called ____________________ . This deficiency is characterized by the four Ds. What are the four Ds?

   a.

   b.

   c.

   d.

6. A niacin deficiency used to occur a lot in the South because people ate a diet that was high in the three Ms. What are these dietary Ms?

   a.

   b.

   c.

7. The function of pyridoxine is to help metabolize fat/protein/carbohydrate.

8. Large intakes of pyridoxine have caused what two toxicities?

   a.

   b.

9. The main function of vitamin B_{12} is to make ______________ ______________ cells. A vitamin B_{12} deficiency is called ______________ anemia because over time the ______________ degenerate and a person dies.

10. A B_{12} deficiency can occur in two ways. Name them.

    a.

    b.

11. The technical name for vitamin C is ______________ ______________. A deficiency of vitamin C is called ______________. List 4 symptoms of this deficiency.

    a.

    b.

    c.

    d.

12. The RDA for vitamin C is ______________ mg/day.

13. To scientifically investigate whether large doses of vitamin C are beneficial in preventing colds, a scientist must conduct ______________ , ______________-______________ experiments.

14. List 4 toxicity symptoms that can occur with excessive vitamin C intake.

    a.

    b.

    c.

    d.

CHAPTER 8

Vitamins — Fat-Soluble

The fat-soluble vitamins consist of vitamins A, D, E and K. When excess fat-soluble vitamins are consumed, the excess is stored in the body, generally in the adipose tissue (fat) or the liver. This storage delays the occurrence of fat-soluble vitamin deficiencies. Generally, it is children who are most at risk for fat-soluble vitamin deficiencies because they do not have the stores that have accumulated in the adult. Fat-soluble vitamins are generally more toxic because excess consumption is stored in the body and not excreted as occurs with water-soluble vitamins. This is especially true for vitamins A and D.

Vitamin A

Vitamin A: Vitamin A was the first vitamin discovered — in the early 1900s. It was shown that rats eating foods in which the fat was removed failed to grow, developed skin problems, went blind and finally died. If the fat was replaced in their diets early in the experiments, the rats recovered completely. However, once blindness occurred because of the deficiency, it was irreversible. Investigators soon discovered that it was not the absence of the fat that was causing the problems, but a factor in that fat. They named this factor a "vitamine" (meaning an amine that was necessary for life).

Soon after, it was discovered that there were other factors essential to life that were found in the water portion of the diet not containing amines. The term vitamin A was used to distinguish the fat-soluble component from the water-soluble vitamin B component.

Retinol (Vitamin A): The chemical name for vitamin A is *retinol.* The requirement for vitamin A for an adult female is *800 retinol equivalents* (RE) per day, while the adult male requires *1000 RE* per day. Men require more vitamin A only because generally they are bigger than women.

We use the term "retinol equivalents (RE)" to specify the vitamin A requirement because different chemical forms of the vitamin A contribute to a person's total vitamin A requirement. Retinol, the most common and active form of the vitamin, is found only in animal products. However, most animal products with the exception of liver are poor sources of vitamin A.

Provitamins

Plant and vegetable products contain the *provitamin* carotene. A provitamin is an inactive form of a vitamin that is found in foods and that the body converts to the active form (in this case retinol). When carotene is absorbed from plant products, some of it is converted to retinol by intestinal cells, thus providing some vitamin A. The rest of the carotene is stored in the fat cells. Unfortunately, it appears that carotene is only converted to vitamin A when it is appears that carotene is only converted to vitamin A when it is initially absorbed. Once it is in the body carotene cannot be converted to retinol. Table 8-1 provides information on the retinol equivalents in some of the better animal (retinol) and vegetable (carotene) food sources.

While orange fruits and vegetables are a good source of carotene, most people are surprised to find that dark green vegetables are also a good source. Chlorophyll, the dark green pigment, masks the presence of carotene in these vegetables. Carotene is always present when chlorophyll is present in foods. The body makes one retinol from every six carotene molecules eaten.

Table 8-1. Vitamin A content of selected foods.

Animal Products	RE/ serving	Vegetable Products	RE/ serving
liver (4 ozs.)	12,000	carrots (1 cup)	2500
milk[1] (1 cup)	100	spinach (1 cup)	2500
egg (1)	80	cantaloupe (1 cup)	1400
beef (4 ozs.)	15	broccoli (1 cup)	700
		cereals[2] (1 cup)	0

1. milk is fortified with vitamin A.
2. some cereals may be fortified with vitamin A.

Vitamin A has three functions in the body.

Vitamin A has three functions in the body: *to promote epithelial cell growth; to promote bone growth;* and *to prevent night blindness.* Epithelial cells are those cells that form a protective layer in the body. These cells are found in the skin, linings of the intestinal tract, lungs, urinary tract, reproductive organs and eyes.

The first sign of a vitamin A deficiency is night blindness. After spending some time in the dark, such as in a movie theater, there is a momentary loss of vision when one is suddenly hit with a bright light. The speed with which a person recovers his vision can indicate that person's vitamin A status. When light hits the eye at night, it causes a change in a chemical in the eye called ***rhodopsin.*** Rhodopsin, which is vitamin A and another chemical, is broken apart when hit with light. Only when the two chemicals rejoin does one's vision return.

More serious vitamin A deficiency symptoms occur as epithelial cell growth is affected. Instead of growing normally, epithelial cells collapse and become ***keratinized*** (Figure 8-1). Keratin is a protein-like substance similar to that found in fingernails. The skin becomes dry, scaly and rough. The taste buds become keratinized leading to a loss of taste and a decrease in appetite. Perhaps the most serious effect is epithelial cell degeneration in the eye. This degeneration, if it develops far enough, leads to a condition called ***xeropthalmia,*** or keratinization of the eye. (Figure 8-2). Xeropthalmia is the leading cause of blindness in children in the world today.

Figure 8-1. Keratinization of the skin in retinol deficiency shown in a female's upper shoulder. (From *Vitamin Manual*, The Upjohn Company, Kalamazoo, MI, 1965.)

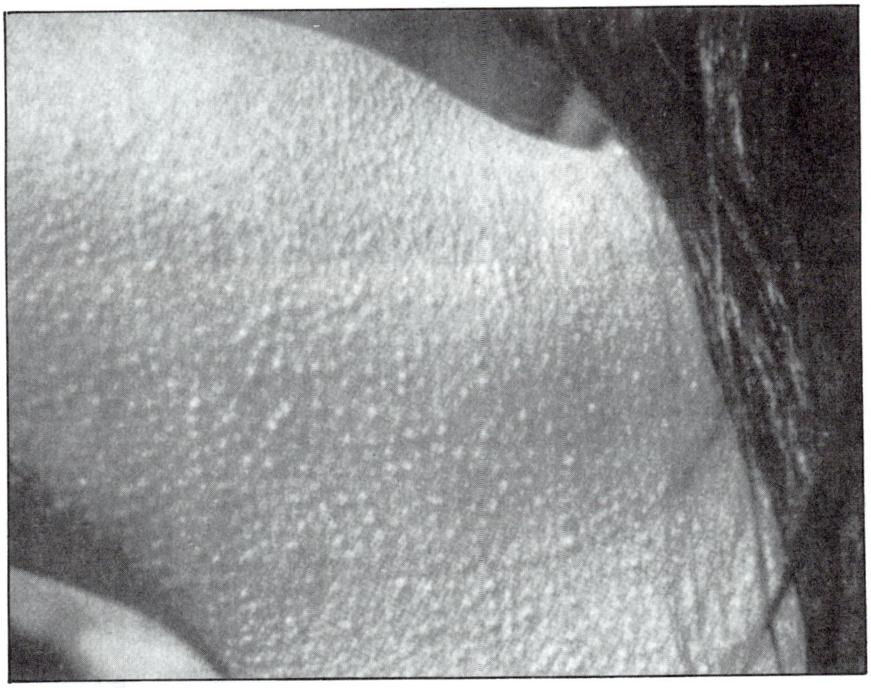

Children are more susceptible to vitamin A deficiency than adults. Adults store any extra vitamin A in their fat cells and liver. If their diet stops meeting their requirement for vitamin A, they can draw on their vitamin A stores. Since children have much less vitamin A accumulated in their tissues, there are frequently inadequate stores to draw from if the diet is limited in vitamin A. Vitamin A deficiency in children is characterized by slow growth, skin problems and in the end, blindness.

Therapeutic uses of Vitamin A

Therapeutic uses of Vitamin A: Vitamin A has for many years been used to reduce the incidence of *severe acne*. Some severe acnes, especially pitting acne, seem to respond to pharmacological doses of vitamin A. Some people require topical applications of the vitamin, while others need to consume the vitamin for it to be effective. We do not know exactly how vitamin A affects acne; but because acne is a disease of epithelial cells, it is probably related to vitamin A's effect on epithelial cell growth.

One of the chemically related forms of vitamin A, retin-A, has recently received much publicity about its anti-aging effects. Retin-A when properly used seems to prevent or reduce skin damage due to sunlight. Moreover, it also seems to revive wrinkled skin. All available evidence suggests that the treatment needs to be continuous for it to be effective. Also, it works best when used in conjunction with sunscreens. Although this treatment seems effective, whether it will really work in the long run remains to be seen.

Figure 8-2. Degeneration of the eye in retinol deficiency. Panel A. Early xeropthalmia in 3 year old Indonesian boy. Panel B. End-stage eye degeneration in 3 year old Tamil Indian girl. (From McLaren, D.S. *Present Knowledge in Nutrition.* 5th edition. The Nutrition Foundation, Washington, D.C., 1984)

Another potential therapeutic function of vitamin A is in the prevention of certain kinds of cancers. Epidemiological (population-based) studies have shown that people with higher levels of retinol (vitamin A) in their blood have a reduced incidence of epithelial cancers (lung, bladder, cervix, etc.). For instance, in one study smokers had one-half the incidence of lung cancers when their blood levels of vitamin A were high as compared to smokers with low blood levels of vitamin A. Animal studies have also shown that increased vitamin A in the diet reduces, but does not entirely eliminate, the occurrence of cancers when the animals are injected with carcinogenic chemicals.

Vitamin A and cancer

Two points need to be made about the relationship between vitamin A and cancer. First, the data only suggest that low levels of dietary vitamin A may lead to an increased risk for developing certain cancers. Neither is there evidence that increased vitamin A intakes will totally prevent cancers. Thus, if one is a smoker, taking extra vitamin A might reduce one's risk of lung cancer, but the risk of developing lung cancer would still be very much greater than in a non-smoker.

A second point to remember is that vitamin A is toxic. For this reason vitamin A supplements are not recommended. Current research is investigating whether carotene supplements, considered non-toxic but able to boost vitamin A levels because some of it is converted to vitamin A, might be beneficial in providing protection against cancer. Many vitamin supplements are now boasting that they also provide carotene.

Toxicity of vitamin A: It was discovered early that continued high doses of vitamin A were toxic. Among the reported toxicities of vitamin A are *headaches, nausea, dry, scaly skin, loss of hair* and *diarrhea*. A much more toxic effect of vitamin A is *birth defects* in babies of mothers taking large doses. For this reason it is not gener-

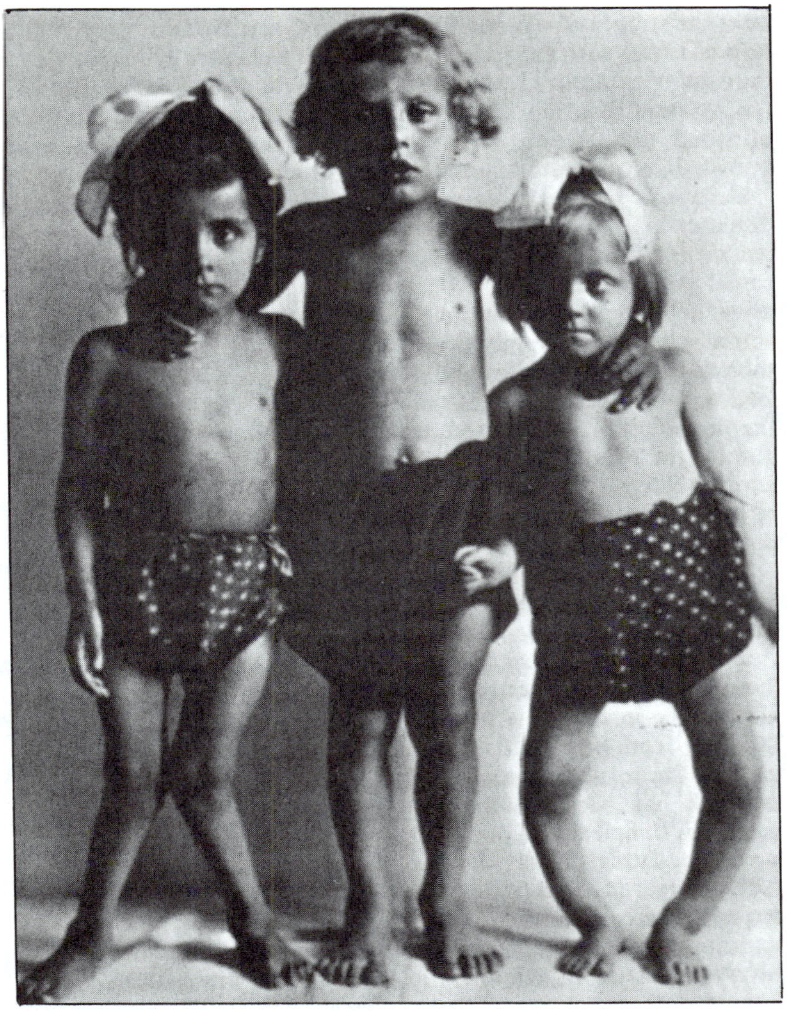

Figure 8-3. Severe rickets in 6 year old girls. The middle child is almost normal. (From Pyke, M. *Man & Food*, McGraw-Hill Book Co., 1965.)

ally prescribed for young, potentially child-bearing women. Current treatments use slightly different chemical forms of the vitamin, modified to be effective but with less toxicity.

Vitamin D

Vitamin D: Vitamin D's main function in the body is to control blood calcium levels. While most people know that the body's calcium is concentrated in the bone, they do not realize the importance of blood calcium. The body maintains blood calcium within very narrow limits because it is necessary for proper *blood clotting*, proper *muscle contraction*, and proper *nerve function*. Every day the body loses about 7% of its blood calcium through the kidneys into the urine. Vitamin D's role is to regulate the loss of calcium from the body and the absorption of dietary calcium.

How Vitamin D Functions: Vitamin D functions in three ways to maintain blood calcium. Vitamin D does this by causing 1) *more calcium to be absorbed from dietary calcium in the intestine* (normally a person only absorbs about 30-40 percent of his dietary calcium); 2) *less calcium to be excreted by the kidneys;* and 3) *calcium to be released from the bone into the blood.* The net results of these changes are blood calcium levels returning to normal and calcium returning to the bone.

A deficiency of vitamin D affects bone development because a person is then unable to absorb enough calcium. In children the deficiency is called *rickets.* (Figure 8-3). Rickets is characterized by soft bones that fail to harden. Children with rickets often exhibit bow-leggedness because their long leg bones cannot adequately support their weight. In the adult vitamin D deficiency is called *osteomalacia.* Osteomalacia is not quite as serious as rickets because the adult already has formed his bones. But osteomalacia can result in a softening of bone over time, as calcium is lost from the bone and not replaced.

Vitamin D deficiencies occur much less often today than they did 40 years ago. Most foods are very poor sources of vitamin D. Only *liver* is a good source of vitamin D. *Eggs* are a fair source of the vitamin. Vitamin D deficiencies were only eliminated with the practice of fortifying *milk and butter* with vitamin D.

Sunlight is a source of Vitamin D.

Another source of vitamin D is sunlight. When the skin is exposed to sunlight, chemical changes occur causing vitamin D to be produced. In areas of the world where people are exposed to sunlight for a significant portion of the year, vitamin D deficiency does not occur. Rickets and osteomalacia only occur in northern areas of the world (areas that do not get much sunlight) and in environments where people are inside much of the time. In these areas of the world it is very important that sufficient vitamin D be consumed in the diet.

In the United States we are concerned about our population's low dietary intake of calcium, especially in women. Lifelong low calcium intakes lead eventually to a deficiency called *osteoporosis* (discussed in Chapter 9). Osteoporosis means literally "porous bone," bone that is very brittle. Since vitamin D increases the absorption of dietary calcium, it might seem reasonable that increases of vitamin D intake will compensate for low calcium intake. However, vitamin D supplements are *not* recommended to overcome the problem of osteoporosis brought about by low dietary calcium intakes.

Vitamin D toxicity: Vitamin D is extremely toxic. The requirement is 400 I.U. (International Units — a way of expressing vitamin D doses). Toxic effects have been observed in some persons receiving as little as 1000 I.U. per day for 1-2 months. This toxicity happens because the extra vitamin D becomes too efficient in its action. Dietary calcium absorption is much increased and kidney excretion is much decreased resulting in *hypercalcemia* (high blood calcium). Hypercalcemia can cause *high blood pressure, kidney stones* and *calcium deposits in soft tissues*. This latter condition can lead to tendon, muscle and nerve problems, eventually resulting in death. So although vitamin D will increase the absorption of dietary calcium, nutritionists do not recommend vitamin D supplements because of their toxicity.

A question often asked is: if vitamin D is toxic, can too much sunlight cause my body to make toxic amounts of the vitamin? The answer is no! As your body is exposed to sunlight, vitamin D is synthesized in the skin. However, after a certain amount of vitamin

D is made, the body stops making it even if it continues to be exposed to sunlight.

Vitamin E

Vitamin E: Vitamin E, another fat-soluble vitamin, is one about which much misinformation exists. The chemical name for vitamin E is *tocopherol*, a word meaning "live birth." The vitamin was so named because in laboratory and farm animals a deficiency in vitamin E causes sterility in male animals and fertility problems in female animals. It seemed reasonable then to assume that vitamin E would also cure many sexual problems in humans. Unfortunately, although vitamin E has been sold as a "love potion vitamin" for many years, it has been proven that the sexual problems associated with vitamin E deficiency in animals do not occur in humans. It is another case of wishful thinking with no scientific foundation.

Another vitamin E deficiency symptom in animals is a muscle deterioration similar to muscular dystrophy in humans. This connection between vitamin E and muscle deterioration has lead to much false hope in people suffering from muscular dystrophy and has made them a target of charlatans selling vitamin E supplements. Vitamin E has no effect on the development of muscular dystrophy in humans. Again, another example of vulnerable people being taken advantage of by fraudulent food claims.

The function of vitamin E is as an *antioxidant*. Antioxidants function to prevent the oxidation (breakdown) of fats. Polyunsaturated fats (those with two or more double bonds) are easily oxidized. Vegetable oils, good sources of polyunsaturated fats, are also good sources of vitamin E. Another good source of vitamin E is wheat germ. However, many commercial sources of wheat germ are de-fatted before they are sold and are consequently not good sources of vitamin E.

There is good evidence that vitamin E also functions as an antioxidant in the body. When fats in the body are oxidized, they produce reactive free radicals. Free radicals tend to be destructive to other components of the cells like membranes and DNA. Vitamin E interacts with free radicals decreasing their toxicity.

Because vitamin E has been shown to protect cells against free radical damage, it has been suggested as an anti-aging and anticancer vitamin. Probably more vitamin E has been sold as a supplement than all the other vitamins combined. It has been advertised as preventing wrinkles because it will protect membranes in the skin against free radical damage. It is also sold in many topical creams like sunscreens supposedly to protect against skin damage. Whether vitamin E has any direct effect on skin damage is questionable. There are no scientific studies that support this contention. However, it does not appear that vitamin E has any major toxic side effects, so persons consuming vitamin E supplements are probably not going to hurt themselves. There is equally no evidence that they are helping themselves.

Extra vitamin E has also been suggested as effective in preventing cancer. Again, the hypothesis is that because vitamin E stops free radical damage to DNA (the first step in cancer occurrence), it will protect against the development of cancer. Unfortunately, research in this area has been unable to prove this hypothesis.

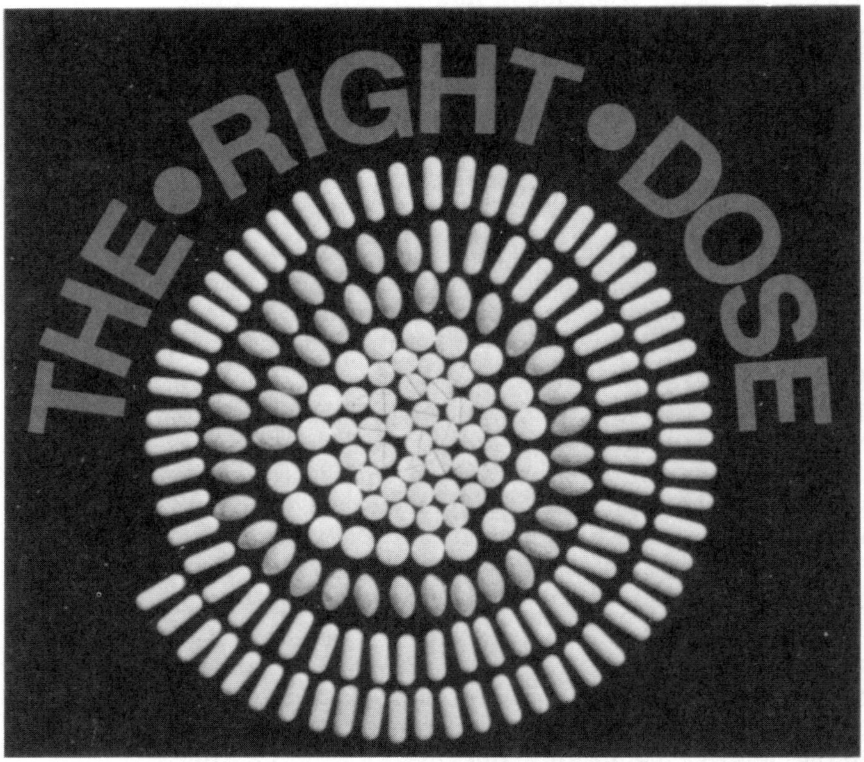

Maria Stenzel/Ann Park

Cher does it. Ronald Reagan, Martina Navratilova, and Victoria Principal do it, too. In fact, 40 percent of Americans take vitamin and mineral supplements. Among the elderly, West Coasters, and dietitians, the percentage is even higher.

Yet in May, 1986, the American Dietetic Association, National Dairy Council, and Food and Drug Administration held a joint press conference to warn the public that supplements can be dangerous.

Are supplements a hazard to health? A new book, *The Right Dose*, offers answers based on fact, not emotion.

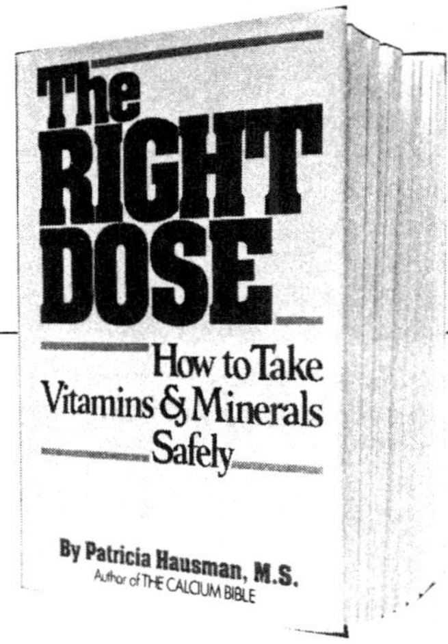

According to author Hausman, *taking supplements can be a low-risk proposition.*

No question about it, too much of some vitamins and minerals can cause harm. It isn't hard to find examples of people who suffered nausea, skin problems, nerve disorders, liver damage, or even death because they carried a good thing too far.

But just how common are such side effects? No one knows precisely, because only as of May, 1986, has FDA asked physicians to report supplement side effects to the agency itself or to a local health department, just as they would drug side effects.

Still, any regular reader of medical journals would have to admit that problems caused by supplements seem to be relatively rare. Considering that generous doses of some vitamins and minerals might help prevent certain cancers, osteoporosis, high blood pressure, and other diseases, it makes sense to examine the evidence carefully, rather than simply dismiss all supplements as dangerous.

The Right Dose: How to Take Vitamins and Minerals Safely is just such an examination. Author Patricia Hausman, a nutritionist who worked for seven years at CSPI, takes the issue of supplement safety head on. While others refuse to recommend supplements because they can't guarantee safety, Hausman has another view:

"I have known people who demanded guarantees that everything they did for better health would make them healthier . . . and do you know what? They found a good way to drive themselves crazy. By expecting guarantees, they set themselves up for disappointment; as soon as an effort toward better health failed to give them everything they had hoped for, they felt like abandoning everything—diet, exercise, and supplements—and leaving their health to chance.

"I have spent enough years in the business of health to know that leaving your health to chance is a lot riskier than taking low-risk efforts to maintain good health. Just think of the impact on our nation's health if all of us who exercise stopped doing so because of the occasional person who suffers a heart attack during physical activity!

"What I have done here, then, is my best job of getting you information to make your supplement program as risk-free as possible. To me, that's what supplement safety is really about."

One other aspect of supplement safety has to be explained at the outset: nutritional individuality. Rarely can scientists identify a dose that adversely affects everyone. Rather, sensitivity to high doses of vitamins and minerals varies—often markedly — from one person to another.

Says Hausman, "I know of no better example [of nutritional individuality] than the case of two 15-year-old brothers, believed to be identical twins, who had both been taking 300,000 I.U. of vitamin A daily for psoriasis. One of the boys developed a severe case of vitamin A overdose, while the other had hardly any symptoms of toxicity at all."

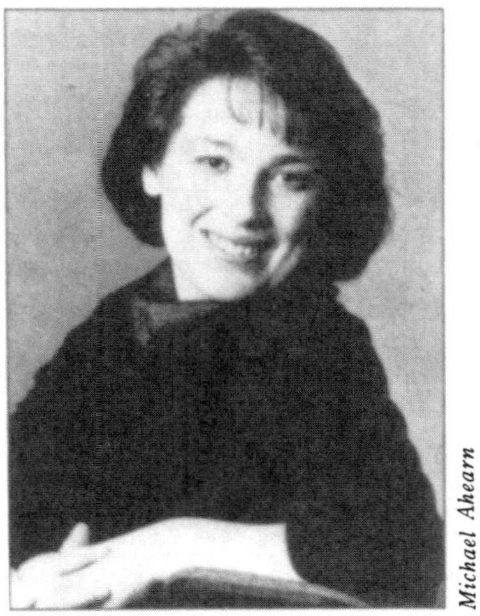

Michael Ahearn

Patricia Hausman *takes the issue of supplement safety head on.*

When nutritionists or physicians report that a vitamin or mineral causes side effects, they aren't asserting that everyone, or even most people, will be afflicted. As with medicines, a "common side effect" is one that may occur in only five percent of patients. Take Hausman's description of the side effects caused by niacinamide, a form of the B-vitamin, niacin.

"The first report comes from a group of dermatologists who treated 204 psoriasis patients with 100 to 3,000 milligrams (mg) of niacinamide daily. Of these 204 subjects, only 8 complained of such symptoms as red patches on the face, dull headache, mild nausea, or flushing. A similar survey among 262 patients who received 3,000 mg daily for 3 to 36 months found that 5 percent of the patients complained of adverse effects."

That said, on with *The Right Dose*. Below, we excerpt sections on topics of special interest. Then, on pages 6 and 7, *NAH* presents a handy chart that summarizes key facts from the text.

Vitamin C: The Hidden Hazard. It all began when a young woman, Elise, found herself suffering from a problem called dental erosion, a condition in which the top surface of the teeth—the enamel—is worn away. Elise sought advice from John L. Giunta, D.M.D., of Tufts University School of Medicine in Boston. Here is her story, as the dentist reported it to the Journal of the American Dental Association:

"A 30-year-old female had requested a second opinion about whether her teeth were eroded and what might be the probable cause. Her dentist had informed her that she had severe dental erosion that required restoration by full crowns on at least 12 teeth. Currently her teeth were painful to brush and she had been told to use a desensitizing toothpaste. When questioned about pills, she admitted taking vitamin supplements including chewable vitamin C tablets."

Dr. Giunta repeated the diagnosis of severe dental erosion given by the first dentist. He told Elise that her daily chewing of multiple vitamin C tablets was

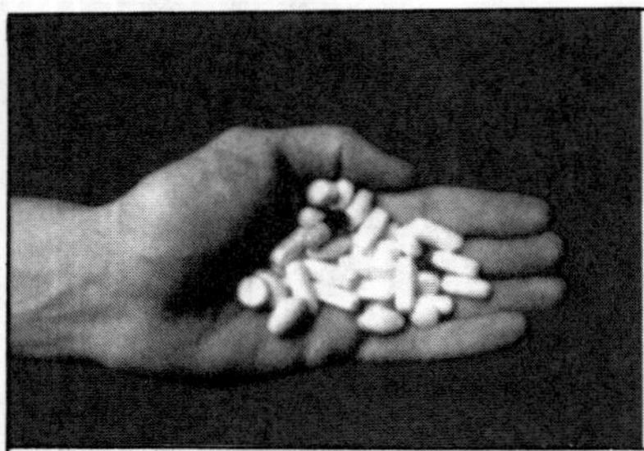

COVER STORY

Supplement safety is complex. Read the following explanations carefully before using this chart, which is based on Patricia Hausman's estimates in *The Right Dose.*

USRDA – The U.S. Recommended Daily Allowance is designed to meet the needs of most healthy people. The Recommended Dietary Allowance (RDA) for your specific sex and age group may be higher or – more commonly – lower than the USRDA.

Adverse Effects – In most cases, these are the effects of taking a supplement at the doses described for several months. Not included are the immediate effects of a much higher dose. "Isolated reports" of adverse effects may not turn out to be valid upon further investigation.

Low-Risk Dose – These doses apply to healthy adults, and include a generous margin of safety.

NUTRIENT	USRDA	ADVERSE EFFECTS
Vitamin A (retinol)	5,000 IU	Toxicity well-documented, usually at doses over 50,000 IU. Symptoms include bone and joint pain, hair loss, itching, dry skin, tender bones, weakness, fatigue.
Thiamine (B-1)	1.5 mg	Two isolated reports of headache, irritability, rapid pulse, trembling, and weakness at doses of 5–10,000 mg.
Riboflavin (B-2)	1.7 mg	None reported.
Niacin (nicotinic acid form)	20 mg	Short-term effects (flushing, rashes, tingling, itching) may occur at doses of 100 mg. Long-term effects include nausea, vomiting, diarrhea, and ulcers at 100–300 mg; jaundice and glucose intolerance at 750 mg or more.
Niacin (niacinamide form)	20 mg	Headache, nausea, and skin blotches at 300–600 mg; fatigue, hives, lightheadedness, sore mouth at 3,000 mg; jaundice, vomiting at 8,000+ mg.
Vitamin B-6	2 mg	Reversible nerve damage (tingling sensation, impaired walking, reaching, sense of touch, vibration, or temperature) at doses of 2,000+ mg.
Folic Acid	400 mcg	May increase zinc excretion above 400 mcg; may mask B-12 deficiency at doses of 1,000+ mcg.
Vitamin B-12	4 mcg	None known.
Pantothenic Acid	10 mg	Isolated reports of diarrhea, water retention, sleepiness, memory loss, depression, nausea at doses of 200–20,000 mg.
Vitamin C	60 mg	Reports of kidney stones, diarrhea, and iron overload at 1,000+ mg; low copper levels at 1,500+ mg; impaired ability to fight bacterial infections and withdrawal symptoms at 2,000 mg; reduced resistance to high altitudes at 3,000 mg.
Vitamin D	400 IU	Toxicity well-documented, usually at doses of 25,000–200,000 IU. Symptoms include nausea, vomiting, loss of appetite, dry mouth, headache, stomach or bone pain, dizziness. Kidney stones and high blood cholesterol may occur at 1,200+ IU.
Vitamin E	30 IU	Isolated reports of blurred vision, fatigue, slowed blood clotting, hormonal changes, raised blood pressure, and allergic skin reactions at doses of 800+ IU.
Calcium	1,000 mg	High blood calcium (nausea, vomiting, high blood pressure, diarrhea, constipation, depression, fatigue, abdominal pain, dry mouth, thirst, excessive urination, muscle wasting, loss of appetite) may occur at doses of 3,000–8,000 mg. Milk-alkali syndrome (resulting in above symptoms plus kidney stones, kidney damage, calcium deposits in the kidney and eye) may occur at doses of 3,000 mg if the source is calcium carbonate.
Chromium	50-200 mcg*	None known, possibly due to lack of use.
Copper	2 mg	None known, possibly due to lack of use.
Iron	18 mg	Constipation, stomach upset may occur at doses of 18+ mg. Iron overload (abdominal or joint pain, bronze-colored skin, fatigue, weight loss, loss of libido, excess thirst and urination, hunger, yeast infections) may occur at doses over 100 mg in healthy people or at lower doses in people with underlying blood or liver disease or genetic predisposition.
Magnesium	400 mg	People taking magnesium-containing antacids, laxatives, or prescription drugs (not supplements) have developed high blood magnesium levels (low blood pressure, drowsiness, slurred speech, unsteadiness, nausea, etc.) at doses of 1,700+ mg.
Selenium	50-200 mcg*	Toxicity well-documented at doses of 2,400–3,000 mcg. Symptoms include brittle hair and fingernails, dizziness, fatigue, garlic odor of breath, jaundice, nausea, diarrhea, and inflamed or discolored skin.
Zinc	15 mg	May lower "good" HDL cholesterol at doses of 80+ mg. Hinders copper absorption at 50+ mg (depending on copper intake). May impair immune response at 150 mg. Nausea, vomiting, diarrhea at doses of 150 mg of zinc sulfate.

* Estimated Safe and Adequate Daily Dietary Intake. No RDA has been set to date.

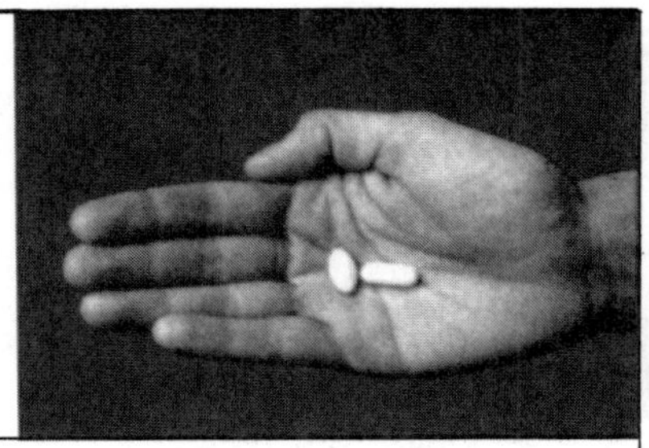

Drug-Nutrient Interactions – These are designed to alert readers to possible problems that should be discussed with a physician. Never compensate for the interaction by taking more of a nutrient or drug without professional advice. In some cases, the interaction may not interfere with nutrient status or drug effectiveness enough to compromise your health. On the other hand, compensating on your own may be dangerous.

The Right Dose, published by Rodale Press, is available in bookstores for $24.95. The comprehensive, 500-page book also includes recipes, food sources, and brand-name supplements for each nutrient. ■

LOW-RISK DOSE	THESE DRUGS MAY INTERFERE WITH NUTRIENT	NUTRIENT MAY INTERFERE WITH THESE DRUGS	SPECIAL PROBLEMS
25,000 IU	Mineral oil, Questran (Cholesterol-lowering drug)	Oral contraceptives	During pregnancy, 18,000+ IU may cause birth defects.
Appears non-toxic.	Antacids, "mercurial" diuretics, barbiturates.	Relaxants sometimes used during surgery.	Some people are allergic to B-1 injections.
Appears non-toxic.	Probenecid, diuretics, Elavil, Tofranil, Thorazine, tetracycline, erythromycin, streptomycin, oral contraceptives.	None known.	Vigorous exercise may double RDA.
100-300 mg	Isoniazid (anti-tuberculosis drug).	Some high blood pressure drugs (ganglionic blockers).	Very high doses may help prevent heart attacks.
100-300 mg	None known.	None known.	None known.
50-100 mg	Oral contraceptives, Seromycin, hydralazine-containing diuretics, Isoniazid, Cuprimine, Depen.	L-dopa, phenobarbital, Dilantin.	According to a preliminary report, 200+ mg may interfere with breast feeding.
400 mcg	Certain antibacterial, anti-convulsant, anti-cancer, anti-tuberculosis, and sulfa drugs; oral contraceptives, cortisone, barbiturates, alcohol.	Anti-convulsants.	Doses of 5,000–10,000 mcg are being tested in cancer prevention studies.
Appears non-toxic.	Alcohol, colchicine, some anti-convulsant and antibacterial drugs.	None known.	Allergy to B-12 injections causes skin problems.
Appears non-toxic.	None known.	None known.	None known.
500-1,000 mg	Barbiturates, oral contraceptives, L-dopa, cortisone, salicylates, aspirin, tetracycline, phenacetin, sulfonamides.	Anti-blood clotting drugs, amphetamines, tricyclic antidepressants.	Chewable tablets may erode tooth enamel.
400-800 IU	Barbiturates, colestipol, Questran, mineral oil phenolphthalein (laxative), cortisone drugs, some anti-convulsants.	Digitoxin, thiazide diuretics.	Infants are more suseptible to toxicity.
400 IU	Mineral oil, iron supplements (in children).	Anti-blood clotting drugs.	Diabetics and thyroid patients should consult a physician.
1,800-2,500 mg	Some diuretics, neomycin, probenecid, Questran, cortisone, mineral oil, phenolphthalein (laxative), lithium, phenobarbital.	Take 2-3 hours apart from tetracycline.	People with a history of kidney stones should consult a physician.
150 mcg	None known.	None known.	None known.
2-3 mg	None known.	None known.	None known.
25-30 mg	Antacids containing carbonates, Questran, Cosmegen, neomycin.	Take 2-3 hours apart from tetracycline.	May impair ability to fight infections that are not being treated with antibiotics.
1,000 mg	Alchohol, probenecid, digitalis, some antibiotics, some anti-convulsants, and some diuretics.	Take 2-3 hours apart from tetracycline.	Kidney patients shouldn't exceed 600 mg.
350-500 mcg	None known.	None known.	Doses of 200 mcg are being tested in cancer prevention studies.
15-25 mg	Some antibiotics, some diuretics, cortisone.	Take 2-3 hours apart from tetracycline.	Sucking on zinc gluconate tablets (to fight colds) may irritate the mouth and distort taste.

Bonnie Liebman compiled this report.

For most people, there is little evidence of kidney stones developing at the higher calcium intakes now recommended to improve bone health.

probably a major cause of her severe dental erosion. She did not believe him, he said, so he set out to convince her otherwise.

Rolling up his sleeves and getting to work, Dr. Giunta first compared the acidity of his own saliva with that of three brands of chewable vitamin C tablets. The tablets were roughly three times as acid. Next he allowed an extracted tooth to sit in a solution of water and an acerola-C wafer—a popular source of chewable vitamin C. Within a few days the tooth enamel became chalky and some of it could be scraped away.

Vitamin D and Heart Health. Recently, nutritionists have seen preliminary evidence that a high intake of vitamin D may be a potential threat to heart health. L.M. Dalderup, M.D., of the Netherlands Institute of Nutrition, has studied the possible effects of vitamin D on blood cholesterol.

In farmers aged 35 to 55, he found that those taking supplemental vitamin D in doses estimated at 700 to 2,500 I.U. daily averaged cholesterol levels of 268 mg (per 100 milliliters of blood). Those *not* taking vitamin D averaged cholesterol levels of 248 mg – substantially lower and more healthful. But there hasn't been any follow-up work to confirm or refute Dr. Dalderup's study.

[However, Victor Linden, M.D., a researcher at the Institute for Community Medicine at the University of Tromso in Norway, has found that retired persons] who suffered heart attacks had had higher vitamin D intakes than those who did not take much vitamin D. According to Dr. Linden, the danger zone seemed to begin at a vitamin D intake of about 1,200 I.U. daily.

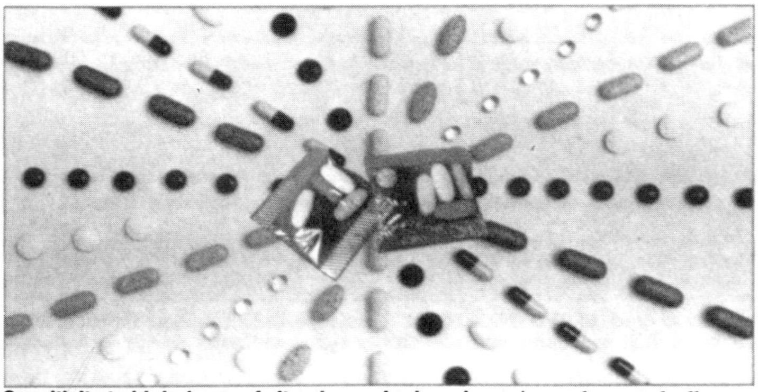

Sensitivity to high doses of vitamins and minerals *varies—often markedly—from one person to another.*

Calcium and Kidney Stones. A 1986 National Institutes of Health panel expressed concern that too much calcium could cause kidney stones in "susceptible people." Those affected often overabsorb calcium; then, having no use for the excess, send it to the kidneys for excretion. In the process, the calcium content of the urine increases, setting the stage for kidney stones.

But for those with normal calcium metabolism and no signs of this disorder, experts say that there is little evidence of kidney stones developing at the higher calcium intakes now recommended to improve bone health. Dr. Robert Heaney, professor of medicine at Creighton University in Omaha, Nebraska, explains that adding an extra 1,000 mg of calcium daily increases the calcium content of the urine by an average of 50 to 70 mg per day in middle-aged and elderly people. That is not an enormous amount.

I see little, if any, reason to suspect that a calcium intake of 2,000 mg per day or less would have much effect on the risk of kidney stones among those with normal calcium metabolism. In fact, I have not found even one report of a woman with normal calcium metabolism who developed kidney stones as a result of calcium supplementation for osteoporosis.

If you are worried that you might be excreting too much calcium without knowing it, ask your doctor for a urinary calcium test. The test is fairly inexpensive and painless, though it does require you to collect your urine for 24 hours.

Zinc: The Copper Robber. The lesson [that zinc impairs the body's ability to absorb copper] was learned the hard way. Physicians had prescribed high doses of zinc in hopes of helping their patients, but several who followed the regimen for more than a year grew increasingly ill. The first case, reported in 1977, concerns a woman referred to as Mrs. L.G.:

"This 59-year-old woman had had several admissions to the hospital for investigation of malabsorption and symptoms of nerve disease. Zinc (150 mg daily) had been prescribed in November, 1975 for non-responsive celiac disease, and the patient had continued to take this oral supplement.

In January, 1977 [14 months later], she was found to have symptoms of severe anemia [extremely low hemoglobin and hematocrit, too few white blood cells, and abnormally low levels of copper in both blood and hair].

She was treated [with blood] transfusion, the zinc supplements were withdrawn, and oral copper given daily. After 12 days, the blood copper had risen [to a normal level]. After 4 weeks she was discharged with a normal blood picture."

Of course [this patient] already had a significant illness. No one could be sure that healthy individuals would react the same way. A few years later, Peter W.F. Fischer, Ph.D., and co-workers at the Canadian Department of Health and Welfare, recruited healthy men and tested their response to daily supplementation with 50 mg of zinc. After six weeks, the men showed signs of declining copper nutrition. It was obvious that high intakes of zinc could inhibit copper absorption in healthy people, too.

Name ______________________________

Section ____________________________

Date ______________________________

Chapter 8
QUESTIONS FOR REVIEW

1. The chemical name for vitamin A is ______________________________ .

2. True vitamin A is found only in animal products. Plant and vegetable products contain a ______________ called ______________ .

3. List the three main functions of vitamin A in the body.

   a.

   b.

   c.

4. The first sign of a vitamin A deficiency is ______________________ blindness. Next epithelial cells become ______________________, or hardened. Finally eye degeneration called ______________________ occurs.

5. Vitamin A has been used therapeutically to treat ______________________ . However, excessive intakes of vitamin A can cause toxic side effects. Name 4 toxic effects.

   a.

   b.

   c.

   d.

6. Vitamin D's function in the body is to regulate blood ______________________ levels. Name two ways vitamin D does this.

   a.

   b.

7. A good food source of vitamin D is ______________________ . Vitamin D can also be made in your body by exposure to ______________________ .

8. A deficiency of vitamin D in children is called rickets whereas in adults the deficiency is called osteomalacia .

9. Vitamin D is more/less toxic than vitamin A.

10. List 4 toxic effects of excessive vitamin D intakes.

    a. death

    b. heart damage

    c. uremia

    d. calcification kidney

11. The main function in the body of vitamin E is as an antioxidant .

12. The best food sources of vitamin E are the vegetable oil wheat germ .

CHAPTER 9

Major Minerals

Minerals are increasingly recognized as being important in both the short- and long-term health of people. Dietary mineral requirements are divided into two classes — the major minerals and the trace elements. The difference between these classes is the amount of the mineral one needs to consume each day. The major minerals are found in the body in relatively large amounts, therefore requiring fairly large daily intakes. Trace elements occur in the body in small amounts, necessitating much smaller intakes. The major minerals to be discussed in this chapter include calcium, sodium and potassium. The trace elements are discussed in Chapter 10.

Table 9-1. Major minerals.

Calcium	Magnesium
Sodium	Phosphorus
Potassium	Sulfur
Chlorine	

Calcium

Calcium is perhaps the most important of the major minerals. As people become elderly, their lifelong calcium intake will determine their quality of life in old age. A lifelong deficiency of calcium leads to a loss of calcium from the bones, a condition called *osteoporosis.* While osteoporosis is especially prevalent in elderly white women, as other population groups (white men, black men and women) live longer, osteoporosis will increasingly affect them.

Functions of Calcium: Most people are aware that calcium is a major mineral in bones. In fact, 99 percent of the calcium in the body is found in the bones. The other 1 percent is found in the blood and soft tissues (muscle and nerves). Table 9-2 provides a list of some critical functions that calcium affects in the soft tissues. These functions affect the ability to sustain life. Too little or too much calcium will interfere with each of the functions listed in Table 9-2. For instance, if blood calcium levels are too high, the body will be unable to clot blood to prevent bleeding. Too little calcium in the blood also affects blood clotting.

Table 9-2. Functions of calcium in the body.

1. Essential for proper blood clotting
2. Essential for transmission of nerve impulses
3. Needed for muscle contraction
4. Essential to control metabolic reactions in all cells

Because of the critical nature of the functions of calcium, the body very tightly regulates the amount of calcium that is found in the blood and soft tissues. Except in some pathological conditions, blood levels of calcium remain very constant. When blood calcium levels start to fall, the body adapts (using vitamin D) by *decreasing excretion of calcium* through the kidneys, *increasing absorption of calcium* from dietary calcium and *removing calcium from the bone.* Through these mechanisms blood calcium levels are returned to normal. When blood calcium levels rise, the body decreases absorption, increases excretion and increases bone calcium.

Every day about 7 percent of the calcium from the blood and soft tissues is lost from the body through the kidneys. In order to keep tissue concentration constant, these losses must be replaced. One way that calcium losses are replaced is through a person's diet. The *calcium requirement* (RDA) for adult men and women is *800 mg/day*. This amount of dietary calcium is needed to replace that lost each day by the body. Nutrition surveys have consistently shown that many women in the United States are consuming much less than the RDA for calcium each day. Men generally consume more calcium per day because they consume more food per day than women, so they are not as much at risk as women. The conclusion from these dietary surveys is that most women in the United States are not meeting their dietary requirement for calcium.

If the diet does not supply the calcium needed to replace daily losses, where does the body get its calcium? *From the BONES!* Whenever calcium intake does not match loss, the body takes calcium from the bones to make up the difference. Over time, if one continues to eat less calcium than is needed, the bones will become depleted of calcium — a condition known as *osteoporosis.*

Osteoporosis means "porous bones."

Osteoporosis literally means "porous bones." The bones become very brittle because of the calcium depletion, and can easily and spontaneously fracture. Osteoporosis can be considered as the endpoint of a lifelong marginal deficiency of calcium. It is a deficiency disease that may take 40 to 50 years to develop.

One of the first signs of osteoporosis is *loss of height*. Calcium loss occurs especially rapidly from the bones of the spinal column. These bones, under pressure from a person's weight, actually lose some of their thickness (see Figure 9-1). This loss results in a loss of height in the person. In elderly ladies, calcium loss from the bones in the neck area of the spinal column can also lead to a condition commonly known as "dowager's hump." Loss of calcium from the spinal column also can lead to *spinal column compression fractures.* Another common and very serious manifestation of osteoporosis is *spontaneous hip and wrist fractures.* It is estimated that over 300,000 spontaneous hip fractures occur each year in the United States. The head of the femur (hip bone) loses calcium, becomes brittle and can no longer carry a person's weight without breaking. Interestingly enough, as many as 15 to 25 percent of people suffering a hip fracture die within six months even if they were in good health prior to its occurrence.

Figure 9-1. Normal and osteoporotic vertebrae. (Source: Courtesy of Anthony A. Albanese, Ph.D., Burke Rehabilitation Center, White Plains, NY.)

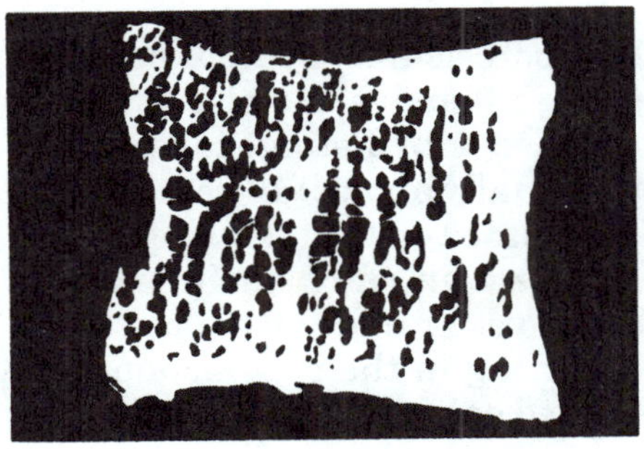

a. normal vertebrae (20 year old female)

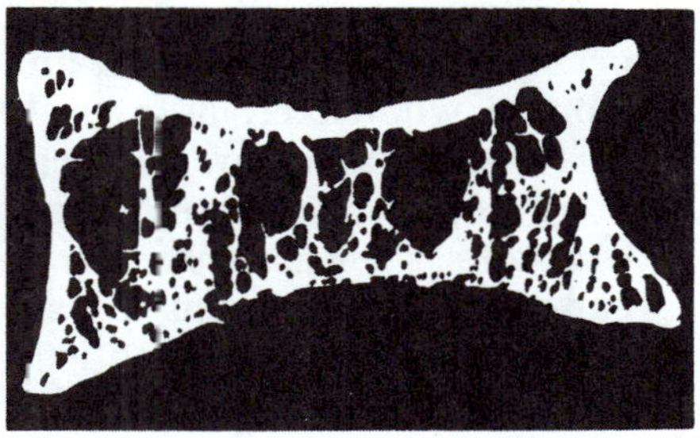

b. osteoporotic vertebrae (60 year old female)

Osteoporosis affects more than twenty million elderly people in the United States today. As people live longer, it will continue to grow as a major health problem. Table 9-3 lists the typical profile of someone suffering from osteoporosis.

Females are afflicted with osteoporosis before males because, besides consuming much less calcium each day than males, female bones are smaller and less dense than male bones. As a result the male can lose more calcium than the female without weakening his bones.

The black population as a whole also has denser bones than does the white population. Thus the white female is most susceptible to osteoporosis with first symptoms occurring at about age 60. Black females and white males (all things being equal) first show symptoms at about age 70 to 75. And black males are chronologically the last, because of their bone density, to exhibit osteoporosis (first symptoms at age 80 to 85).

Table 9-3. Typical osteoporosis profile.

- female
- white
- inactive
- lifelong low calcium intake
- multiple pregnancies during lifetime
- smokes cigarettes
- estrogen-deficient after menopause

Exercise also affects the course of the disease. In young people many studies have shown that exercise will increase the density of one's bone. By developing denser bones when a person is young, the occurrence of osteoporosis when that person ages will be delayed.

Exercise builds denser bones.

Exercise is also of benefit to the elderly because it slows down the loss of calcium from the body and therefore the loss of calcium from the bone. It appears that exercise works in three ways to delay the onset of osteoporosis. Exercise also causes *less calcium to be lost* by way of the kidney from the body each day. And finally, exercise causes an *increase in bone calcium,* making bones denser and stronger.

Estrogen

Exercise can be overdone. Osteoporosis-like symptoms have occurred in young women undergoing intensive exercise. In these women, when exercise (usually combined with dieting) causes body fat levels to fall below a critical level (usually about 9-10 percent), the body stops producing estrogen. As discussed on the following pages, estrogen is necessary for the body to retain calcium. Intensively exercising young women lose calcium very rapidly from the body, similar to the accelerated losses occurring in the post-menopausal woman. The combination of accelerated calcium loss and intensive exercise has recently resulted in documented cases of spontaneous hip fractures in young women.

Another important factor in the development of osteoporosis in women is the lack of estrogen after menopause. Estrogen causes the body to retain calcium. After menopause, when women stop producing estrogen, calcium is lost from the body much faster than before menopause. As a result bone calcium loss increases dramatically after menopause, accelerating the course of osteoporosis. It is uncertain whether taking calcium supplements will completely slow the loss of calcium to pre-menopausal levels. Instead estrogen replacement therapy is often indicated as a means of slowing bone calcium loss after menopause. In studies where very small levels of estrogen were given, calcium loss was reduced to pre-menopausal levels. The use of estrogen is controversial because doses larger than those used to prevent osteoporosis may increase the risk of cancer.

Absorption and Excretion

Factors that Affect Calcium Absorption and Excretion: The amount of calcium that is absorbed from the diet can vary depending on many diet and physiological factors. This variability in the absorption of calcium is called "bioavailability." Likewise, there appear to be many factors that affect the loss of calcium through the kidneys. Sometimes only very small changes in absorption and excretion will produce major effects over time. This is especially true for many women whose calcium intake is very small. Since the body will use the bone's calcium to replace any deficit, factors that decrease absorption or increase excretion of calcium will accelerate the occurrence of osteoporosis. Any factors that will increase the absorption of calcium from the diet or decrease its loss from the body will delay the onset.

The body absorbs only about 30 to 40 percent of one's dietary intake of calcium. Some factors that increase the absorption of dietary calcium are *vitamin D, exercise, dietary lactose* (associated with milk) and the *calcium-to-phosphorus ratio of the diet.* Generally, Americans eat a diet that is low in calcium and high in phosphorus. The high phosphorus intake (found in high protein foods) reduces the body's ability to absorb calcium. All other factors being equal, a person eating a high-protein diet would need more calcium (because less would be absorbed) than a person eating a low-protein diet. A cause of osteoporosis in women in the United States may be the combination of marginal calcium intake and high-protein diets. As will be mentioned in the next section, high-protein intakes also cause the body to excrete more calcium each day.

The body loses about 7 percent of its free calcium per day. Factors that can increase the excretion of calcium (by the kidneys) include low estrogen levels, low vitamin D levels, inactivity, cigarette smoking and high dietary protein intakes. Research suggests that if Americans ate a low-protein diet the requirement for calcium would be much less than it is. High-protein diets cause more calcium to be excreted by the kidney.

Your bones are a calcium bank.

What can be done to stop osteoporosis? Two courses of action are possible. Young people should attempt to increase the amount of calcium in their bones. Think of your bones as a calcium bank. The more calcium deposited in your bones while you are young, the longer it will take to deplete them as you age. Until about the age of 30, bone density can increase. The two best ways to increase bone density are to eat dietary calcium and to undertake moderate exercise. Moderate exercise should be an integral part of one's lifestyle as exercise will cause more calcium to be retained by the body, resulting in stronger, denser bones. Even very small-boned women can increase their bone density if they increase their calcium intake and exercise.

After age thirty or so, most research shows that it is not possible to increase the calcium in the bones. People over age thirty should attempt to slow the rate of calcium loss from the bones by increasing their calcium intake and by moderately exercising — the same way one increases bone density when one is younger. Older women who are losing significant amounts of bone after the onset of menopause should consider estrogen replacement therapy. Physicians now have ways to measure bone density and therefore can monitor changes over time.

Calcium sources are mainly dairy products.

Sources of calcium: Few foods are good sources of calcium. The best sources of calcium are milk and other dairy products. Milk provides about 250 mg per 8-ounce glass, a little less than 1/3 of one's requirement per day. About 3 ounces of cheese will also provide about 200 mg of calcium. The only other significant source of calcium in the diet is green leafy vegetables. Spinach, kale, mustard greens and turnip greens all provide about 100 mg per serving (1 cup). Most other components of the diet contain small amounts of calcium, but only milk products and dark green leafy vegetables are concentrated sources of calcium.

Think about your diet. Do you consume 3 glasses of milk per day? How about 2 glasses of milk and one serving of cheese, yogurt or ice cream? This latter example provides the same amount of calcium but with more kilocalories. Many people do not consume any milk products daily. If you consume no milk products, it will be very difficult for you to meet your calcium requirement unless you eat about 8 to 10 servings of spinach or greens daily. Even if one consumes some milk products, it is still difficult to consume one's needed calcium.

Since it is difficult to eat enough dietary calcium, many calcium supplements are being advertised. If you suspect that your diet is not meeting your calcium needs, then a supplement may be advisable. However, if you do decide to take a calcium supplement, *at most all you need is a daily supplement that contains 1000 mg. You absolutely should not consume more than 1000 mg of calcium in supplement form per day.*

Table 9-4. Average calcium content of selected foods.

Food	(serving size)	Calcium/Serving
Whole Milk	(8 oz.)	280 mg
Skim Milk	(8 oz.)	300 mg
Cheese, Cheddar	(1 oz.)	210 mg
Ice Cream	(1 cup)	150 mg
Yogurt	(1 cup)	275 mg
Broccoli	(1 cup)	150 mg
Greens, turnip	(1 cup)	99 mg
Bread, white	(1 slice)	20 mg
Apple	(large)	10 mg

Adapted from *Food Values of Portions Commonly Used.* (ed. C.F. Church and H.N. Church) J.P. Lippincott Co., New York, 1975.

Excessive calcium consumption is associated with some toxic symptoms. The major symptoms of calcium toxicity are *excessive bleeding* and *softening of the bones.* These symptoms can occur in persons consuming about 10,000 mg of calcium per day over time (or about 10 times the amount in one calcium supplement). Unfortunately, some people believe that "if one pill is good, 10 or 20 are better." So while calcium toxicity is rare, it still can occur in persons taking too many calcium supplements.

Most experts recommend supplements that contain calcium carbonate. However, research has shown that there is very little difference in the absorption of calcium in supplements regardless of the source. You may want to buy whichever source of calcium is the least expensive.

Sodium

Sodium: Sodium is the mineral that primarily controls water balance in the body. Most of the body's sodium is found in the blood. Water intake (as indicated by thirst) and water losses (excretion through the kidney as urine) are controlled to a large extent by the body sensing blood sodium levels. When blood sodium levels rise, such as occurs during exercise when water is lost from the body as sweat, the body tries to retain water by increasing the concentration of the urine. (Notice how much more concentrated your urine is after exercise). The increase in blood sodium also triggers a thirst mechanism, increasing your desire to drink.

When blood sodium levels are less concentrated than normal, this signals the body to release water by increasing the volume of dilute urine. Caffeine and alcohol act as *diuretics*. This means that they cause the kidney to release water, increasing urine output. People are often very thirsty after a night of drinking because the alcohol caused dehydration. The body senses the more concentrated blood sodium levels and activates the thirst mechanism.

Salt is the major source of sodium.

One of the dietary goals is to reduce one's sodium intake (or salt intake, as a person's major dietary source of sodium is salt). Whenever you eat foods that contain a lot of salt, blood sodium levels rise. An increase in blood sodium levels, as opposed to their concentration, causes the body to retain water. This usually only happens until the kidney is able to excrete the extra sodium and the extra water into the urine. Then a person's blood volume and sodium levels return to normal.

Table 9-5. Sodium content of selected foods.

Food (serving size)		Sodium/Serving
Cheese, American processed	(1 oz.)	325 mg
Cheese, Cheddar	(1 oz.)	200 mg
Cheese, Swiss	(1 oz.)	250 mg
Bologna	(1 slice)	400 mg
Pickle, Dill	(large)	1450 mg
Tomato	(1 small)	3 mg
Tomato Juice	(1 cup)	400 mg
Tomato soup, canned	(1 cup)	900 mg

Adapted from *Food Values of Portions Commonly Used.* (ed. C.F. Church and H.N. Church) J.P. Lippincott Co., New York, 1975.

About 20 percent of the U.S. population is unable to excrete the excess sodium. When these people consume a lot of sodium (salt) in their diet, they tend to retain sodium and as a result retain water. This causes *hypertension* or *high blood pressure*.

High blood pressure is one of the three major risk factors for heart disease and stroke. Thus, any reduction that occurs in blood pressure will reduce the risk of these diseases occurring. Research has shown that reducing one's salt consumption will lower blood pressure. This is especially true in that percentage of the population that tends to retain sodium.

The typical American diet contains a lot of salt. It is estimated that the average American's *non-discretionary* salt intake is at least 3-5 grams per day. Non-discretionary salt is the salt naturally occurring in your food or the salt that is added to food products during processing and/or during institutional cooking (restaurants, etc.). *Discretionary salt* is that salt added from the salt shaker or the salt added during the cooking of foods at home. Estimates of average discretionary salt usage range from 4 to 10 grams per day, Thus, average total salt intake ranges from 6 to perhaps 15 grams each day.

The easiest way to reduce one's salt intake is to leave the salt shaker on the table. By not salting one's food and not using salt in home cooking, a person could cut his salt consumption at least in half. Research has shown that even modest reductions in salt consumption will lower blood pressure. For those persons with more serious hypertension, both discretionary and non-discretionary salt intake should be reduced. Luckily, food manufacturers have begun to produce low-salt or salt-free pruducts. Also, it is now required by law that the sodium content of a food be listed on the nutritional label. The Food and Drug Administration has recently developed guidelines to clarify sodium claims on products (Table 9-6). Now products can only make sodium claims if they meet specific guidelines.

Table 9-6. Sodium labeling of food products.

A. Sodium Free — contains less than 5 mg sodium per serving
B. Very Low Sodium — contains between 5-35 mg sodium per serving
C. Low Sodium — contains between 35-140 mg sodium per serving
D. Reduced Sodium — 75% reduction in sodium as compared to original product

Potassium

Potassium: Potassium, another major mineral, has a role that opposes sodium. Unlike sodium, which functions outside the cell, (i.e., regulating water in the blood), potassium's major function is to regulate processes inside the cell. Potassium is especially important in controlling muscle contractions. When the body becomes depleted of potassium (as can occur with excessive vomiting or overuse of laxatives in the anorexic), muscle contractions can become erratic. Certain medicines (diuretics) and some diet plans for rapid weight loss also cause the body to lose potassium. In some cases potassium loss can be so great that the heart (your body's most important muscle) stops beating.

Potassium may also function to control blood pressure. The average American diet is low in potassium and high in sodium. Research has shown that potassium counteracts the effect of high sodium diets by lowering blood pressure. When people with essential hypertension consume extra potassium, often their blood pressure decreases.

Sources of potassium are plant and vegetable products.

The best food sources of potassium are plant and vegetable products. Bananas, oranges, potatoes and peanuts (including peanut butter) are especially good sources of potassium. Remember that fresh fruits and vegetables, while being good sources of potassium, also contain very little sodium (Table 9-7). "Lite" salt formulations are another good source of potassium as they are made by replacing much of the sodium with potassium. The best way to increase one's potassium is by increasing one's consumption of fresh fruits, vegetables and whole grains as this also lowers one's intake of sodium.

Table 9-7. Comparative content of sodium and potassium in foods.

Food	(sodium/serving)	Potassium/Serving
Apple (1 small)	1 mg	110 mg
Banana (1 medium)	2 mg	440 mg
Orange (1 medium)	2 mg	400 mg
Potato, baked (medium)	4 mg	500 mg
Peanuts, roasted, unsalted (3.5 oz)	2 mg	740 mg
Peanut butter (1 tbls)	18 mg	125 mg

Adapted from *Food Values of Portions Commonly Used.* (ed. C.F. Church and H.N. Church) J.P. Lippincott Co., New York, 1975.

One should not consume potassium supplements except under a physician's direction because as with many other nutrients there may be toxicities associated with excessive potassium.

To summarize, this chapter has discussed the role of three major minerals — calcium, sodium and potassium — in health. Calcium, a nutrient which is generally consumed in less than optimal amounts by Americans, affects the occurrence of osteoporosis. Sodium, a nutrient that is consumed in excess by Americans, contributes to hypertension. Potassium may diminish the increase in blood pressure caused by the large intakes of sodium.

Tackling High Blood Pressure

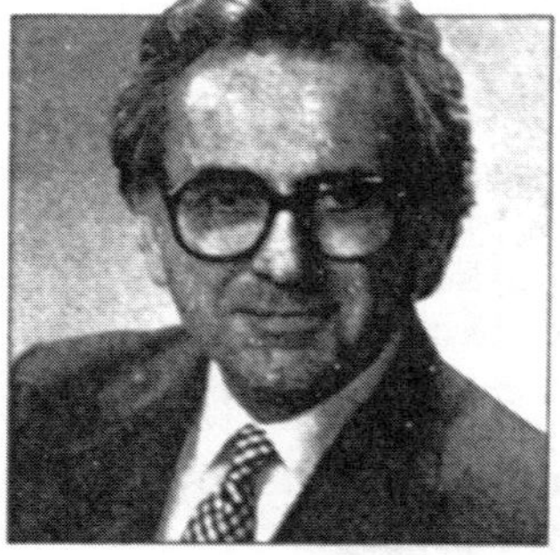

Norman Kaplan

Few people know as much about high blood pressure as Norman Kaplan, Head of the Hypertension Section at the University of Texas Southwestern Medical School. Kaplan has written more than 300 scientific papers, and he served on the Third and Fourth Joint National Committees on the Detection, Evaluation, and Treatment of High Blood Pressure. His books include Clinical Hypertension, Prevention of Coronary Heart Disease, Prevent Your Heart Attack, *and* Hypertension. *His latest book,* Travel Well, *co-authored by his wife, Audrey, lists restaurants in 44 cities that will help diners keep their blood pressure and cholesterol down.*

NAH*'s Bonnie Liebman spoke with him from CSPI's office in Washington, D.C.*

Q: In the past, doctors were concerned that high blood pressure was going untreated. Are people now being *over*treated?

A: Yes. To begin with, the diagnosis is being made too quickly, and many people are being diagnosed as having high blood pressure when, in fact, they don't. In a recent study, researchers used automatic monitors to measure the blood pressures of almost 300 hypertensives. The monitoring was done outside the doctor's office, while the people were working, riding subways, and going about their daily lives in New York City. The study showed that about 20 percent of them only had high blood pressure when it was measured in the doctor's office. A lot of hypertensive people probably only have what we call "office hypertension."

Q: How can people tell if they really have high blood pressure?

A: People should be aware that a single blood pressure measurement isn't enough. They should get multiple readings. We're also doing a lot more home blood pressures. *Consumer Reports* (August, 1987) did a story on devices that measure blood pressure at home. I firmly believe it's a technique we ought to be pressing people to perform.

DRUGS

Q: Once the diagnosis is made, do physicians feel compelled to treat high blood pressure?

A: They often do. Most physicians say, "why bother to make a diagnosis if you're not going to do something?" Doctors are simply trying to help people reduce their risk of heart attack and stroke, but they often don't realize that most people with fairly mild hypertension are not at that big a risk. In fact, physicians often could simply monitor the patient's blood pressure and use dietary approaches before they jump to medication.

Q: Why are some doctors so eager to prescribe drugs?

A: A lot depends on the physician's and the patient's time and energy. It's easier to write out a prescription and give it to the patient than to spend a half hour discussing why he or she needs to go on a diet, start exercising, or cut back on alcohol.

Also, the doctor knows the medication will work. That's not necessarily true for sodium restriction or cutting back on drinking. Not all people who make those changes have a significant fall in blood pressure. So the assumption is that we can't depend on these non-drug approaches, while we know medication will be effective.

Q: Don't drugs have adverse effects?

A: We're now increasingly aware of the hidden toxicities of drugs. Diuretics are the largest selling high blood pressure drug. Over fifty million prescriptions were written last year. We know that chronic use of diuretics may raise cholesterol for a significant number of patients by five to ten percent. That's about 20 points.

Also, diuretics cause blood sugar levels to become elevated in some people and potassium to fall in about one-third of patients. So we have a number of problems with diuretics—which is not to say they should be thrown out. Rather, we should use them more judiciously. For example, we used to give up to 200 mg. of the most common form of diuretic, hydrochloro-

"We're now aware of the hidden toxicities of drugs."

thiazide. Now we know that one-twentieth, or 10 mg., may be enough.

Q: What about other blood-pressure-lowering drugs?

A: Over thirty million prescriptions for beta-blockers were written last year. These medications can cause HDL ["good"] cholesterol to decline.

So while we're lowering blood pressure, we're creating conditions that increase another risk factor. It doesn't happen to every patient, but it can happen, and a lot of people are taking these drugs without being aware of the potential problems.

Picking Up Potassium

Most people eat only about 2,500 mg. of potassium per day. Our blood pressures might be lower if that number were closer to 4,000 mg. Use the chart below to add potassium-rich foods (especially low-fat, high-fiber fruits, vegetables, and beans) to your diet.

	Potassium (mg.)
Dairy Products	
Yogurt, plain, low-fat (1 cup)	531
Milk, 1% fat (1 cup)	381
Fruits and Fruit Juices	
Avocado (½ medium)	602
Watermelon (1/16)	560
Banana (1 medium)	451
Cantaloupe (¼ melon)	412
Orange juice, frozen (6 oz.)	354
Raisins (¼ cup)	308
Grapefruit juice (6 oz.)	284
Orange (1 medium)	237
Apple juice (6 oz.)	222
Pear (1)	208
Beans (cooked, 1 cup)	
Soybeans	886
Lentils	731
Red kidney beans	713
Split peas	710
White navy beans	669
Black-eyed peas	476
Meat, Fish & Poultry (cooked, 4 oz.)	
Rainbow trout	723
Halibut	657
Pork, average, trimmed	416
Beef, average, trimmed	401
Flounder	392
Turkey, skinless	340
Chicken, skinless	277
Vegetables (cooked)	
Potato (1 large)	844
Squash, acorn (½ cup)	446
Spinach (½ cup)	419
Sweet potato (1)	397
Rutabaga (½ cup)	344
Squash, butternut (½ cup)	290
Brussels sprouts (½ cup)	247
Carrot, raw (1)	233
Zucchini (½ cup)	228
Peas (½ cup)	217
Cauliflower (½ cup)	200

SODIUM

Q: How effective are non-drug treatments, such as low-salt diets?

A: About 50 percent of the people who cut their sodium in half will have a significant fall in blood pressure. Studies find an average drop of about 5-over-4 mm. of mercury (Hg). That's not a big-league fall, but it's significant.

Three-fourths of all people with high blood pressure have mild hypertension—that is, their blood pressure is between 140 to 150 over 90 to 100 mm. Hg. It's these people who ought to try non-drug therapies, because they're the ones who are often going to have enough of a drop to bring their blood pressure down to normal.

Q: Does a young person with normal or low blood pressure have to worry about sodium?

A: If we could be sure they wouldn't develop hypertension, no. If someone in your family has hypertension or if you're overweight, we know you have a significantly greater likelihood of developing hypertension. But we have no good marker to determine who is sodium-insensitive and therefore doesn't have to worry. That's why a population-wide push to cut down on sodium makes the most sense.

Q: What did we learn from the recent "Intersalt" study that compared sodium intakes and blood pressures in several countries?

A: Those who don't like sodium say it proves their point. Those who like sodium say the same.

The study found that there was no difference in blood pressure between populations that consumed a lot or a little sodium. But that was only true after researchers excluded populations that consumed very little sodium, and I don't think that's fair.

What's more, in populations with higher sodium intakes, blood pressures rose more steeply as people aged. In populations with lower sodium intakes, blood pressures didn't rise as high as people got older.

If blood pressure didn't rise with age in the U.S., hypertension would no longer be a major public health problem. In other words, if we consumed less sodium, it *would* make a difference.

The study does suggest that beyond a threshold of two grams [2,000 mg.] of sodium per day, it probably doesn't matter how much you consume. Now, that's true as far as the *development* of hypertension is concerned, and if you look at *large populations*. On the other hand, if you cut an *individual's* intake down from four grams to two, in many cases you will see a positive effect.

ILLUSTRATION: LOEL BARR

> "About 50 percent of the people who cut their sodium in half will have a significant fall in blood pressure."

POTASSIUM

Q: Is potassium getting too little credit for its role in lowering high blood pressure?

A: Potassium does need more attention. We don't have as much evidence for potassium as for sodium, but there are a number of good studies showing that adding about 2 to 3 grams of potassium to a diet that already has about that much potassium can lower blood pressure by 3 to 5 mm. Hg. Louis Tobian at the University of Minnesota has shown that potassium protects against kidney damage and strokes in animals.

I tell people not to take potassium tablets, but to eat more natural, unprocessed foods—anything that comes out of the ground. Nature never intended us to eat a lot of sodium, because all foods—fruits, vegetables, meats, grains—are low in sodium. Only when they're processed do we leach out the potassium and add the sodium.

CALCIUM & MAGNESIUM

Q: How good is the evidence that calcium lowers blood pressure?

A: It's a major controversy. In most studies, adding 800 to 1,500 mg. of calcium lowers blood pressure by about 5 mm. Hg in one-third or less of the patients. No one has found that all patients respond.

David McCarron, of the Oregon Health Sciences University in Portland, is calcium's major advocate, and his research is heavily supported by the National Dairy Council.

But I don't think giving calcium supplements has been documented as useful in lowering blood pressure.

As for epidemiological evidence, most of the careful analyses of the National Health and Nutrition Examination Survey data say low calcium intakes are not linked to high blood pressure, except for black males.

Furthermore, we have no rationale that would explain why more calcium would lower blood pressure. On the contrary, we expect calcium to tighten blood vessels and contract the heart.

The only exception may be people who excrete extra calcium in their urine. That may lower blood calcium, which would increase the levels of parathyroid hormone, which in turn could raise blood pressure.

Giving these people calcium might do something. But they probably comprise no more than 30 percent of those with high blood pressure. And keep in mind that extra calcium could increase the risk of kidney stones in people who are already excreting calcium in their urine.

Q: Is there any evidence that magnesium lowers blood pressure?

A: In well-controlled studies, magnesium doesn't seem to have an effect.

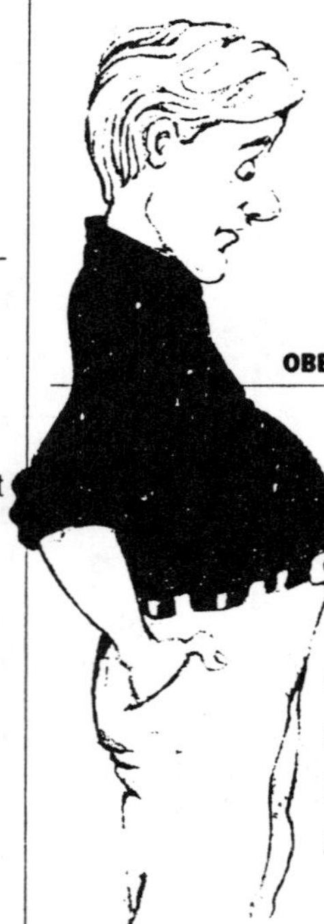

OBESITY

> *Being even slightly overweight can increase risk.*

Q: How important is the link between obesity and high blood pressure?

A: Being even slightly overweight can increase the risk of hypertension, especially for the upper-body obese—those people with excess fat mainly in their abdomen and chest. The simplest way to tell if you've got upper-body obesity is to divide your waist measurement by your hip measurement. If the number is higher than 0.85, you're at risk.

I'm a good example. Even though I haven't gained much weight, and I'm not overweight, over the years my weight has shifted to my waist. My ratio is 0.94, which puts me above the risky level.

I never thought my waist was a health problem, only a social one. I've taken it as a personal challenge to start a better diet and exercise program.

Q: Why should a paunch put you at greater risk than chubby thighs or hips?

A: Abdominal fat is metabolically different than fat that's stored in the thighs and hips. Lower-body fat is largely inactive, except during pregnancy and lactation, when the thighs serve as a depot for fat stores that are used to make milk.

In contrast, upper body fat is active—that is, it is more readily released from the cells into the bloodstream, where it can clog arteries. The fat can also enter the liver, where it may interfere with the body's ability to get rid of insulin. That increases insulin levels in the blood, which turns out to raise blood pressure.

ALCOHOL AND FIBER

Q: How does alcohol affect blood pressure?

A: Social drinking can raise blood pressure. One or two drinks a day is okay, but with more than two drinks—about an ounce of alcohol—you begin to see effects on blood pressure.

Q: What about polyunsaturated fats or fiber?

A: We don't have enough data to say they lower blood pressure. My advice is to eat less saturated fat and more fiber, but for other reasons. ☐

Name ____________________

Section ____________________

Date ____________________

Chapter **9**

QUESTIONS FOR REVIEW

1. The calcium requirement for a woman in the United States is currently ________ mg/day. Most women meet/do not meet this requirement.

2. *Osteoporosis* literally means ______________ ______________ .

3. A profile of the typical person at risk for developing osteoporosis is:

   a.

   b.

   c.

   d.

4. Variability in the absorption of dietary calcium is called ______________ . List 4 factors that increase the absorption of dietary calcium and list three factors that decrease the absorption.

Increase	Decrease
a.	a.
b.	b.
c.	c.
d.	

5. Milk provides about ________ mg of calcium per 8-ounce glass, while green leafy vegetables provide about ________ mg of calcium per serving.

6. If you do decide to take a calcium supplement the most you should take in any day is ________ mg.

7. List two symptoms of excessive calcium intake.

   a.

   b.

8. The technical name for high blood pressure is ___Hypertensia___ .

9. A major mineral in the diet that contributes to high blood pressure is ___Sodium___, while a mineral that may protect against high blood pressure is ___Potassion___ .

10. Salt that is added to one's food at the table, or in cooking is called ___discre___ salt. Salt that is in foods that one has no control over (such as salt added to aid processing) is called ___nondiscre___ .

CHAPTER 10

Minerals — Trace Elements

The trace elements are those minerals that are needed by the body in very minute amounts. However, the trace elements are not any less important than the major minerals. In fact, often people's diets are more lacking in the trace elements than the major minerals. Table 10-1 lists all of the trace elements known to be essential to man. People are often surprised that some toxic elements such as arsenic and lead are required by man. Even though many trace elements are toxic in large doses, humans do need them in very small amounts. The requirement for most of the trace elements is so small that any food intake at all will provide enough to meet one's need. Discussed in this chapter will be iron, zinc and iodine, three trace elements which humans may not always consume in adequate quantities.

Table 10-1. Trace elements required by man.

Iron	Silicon	Lead
Zinc	Selenium	Tin
Iodine	Manganese	Arsenic
Fluorine	Molybdenum	Vanadium
Copper	Nickel	Cobalt
Chromium		

Iron: Many people, most notably females and children, do not consume enough iron in their diets. Nutritional surveys have shown that about 1/3 of the children (ages 2 to 9 years) in this country consume less than 70 percent of their RDA for iron. These same surveys (Table 10-2) also point out that more than 50% of the adolescent girls and 50% of the adult women in this country consume less than 70% of their RDA for iron. Remember, a nutrient's RDA is the intake of that nutrient necessary to meet the needs of almost all (95%) of the population. So an RDA is only a rough approximation of an individual's need. Yet if a person is consistently consuming less than 70% of his RDA of a nutrient, this is a strong indication that intake of this nutrient is less than optimal. *Iron*

Table 10-2. Iron status of American people: Results of the HANES survey.

Group	Percent consuming 100% of RDA for iron	Percent consuming 70% of RDA for iron
Children	38%	64%
Adolescents		
Boys	36%	74%
Girls	18%	45%
Adults		
Men	88%	98%
Women	18%	44%

Women and children need more iron.

Why is it so difficult for children and women to get enough iron in their diets? There are two reasons. First, both of these population groups have an *increased need for iron*. Children, because they are growing, need to increase their blood volume. Women need more iron than men because they must replace blood that is lost during menstruation. The major function of iron is to *make hemoglobin, a necessary component of red blood cells. When blood needs increase, iron needs also increase.* Secondly, *few foods are good sources of iron.* The average diet provides only 6 mg of iron per 1000 kcals. The *RDA for men is 10 mg/day,* while the *RDA for women is 15 mg/day.* This means that the average woman needs to consume about 3000 kcals per day to meet her iron requirement, whereas the average man needs to consume only about 1800 kcals per day. How many women consume 3000 kcals per day? Very few, so most women have a very difficult time meeting their requirement for iron through the diet.

Table 10-3 shows the major dietary sources of iron. Besides liver only beef and fortified cereals are good sources of iron. Even so, for a female to meet her iron need, she would have to consume about 2.5 servings of liver or about 6 hamburger patties daily. Whole grains, although fair sources of iron, present the body with iron in a form that is hard to absorb.

Table 10-3. Food sources of iron.

Food	Iron content (mg/serving)
Liver (4 ozs)	8
Beef (4 ozs)	3
Cereal, fortified (1 cup)	2.5
Chicken (4 ozs)	1.8
Bread, whole grain (2 slices)	1.4

Iron Bioavailability: Another factor that affects a person's iron status is *iron bioavailability*. Bioavailability is a term referring to the amount of a mineral in the diet that is absorbed by the body. As previously discussed in the chapter on calcium, certain dietary factors or physiological conditions affect the percentage of calcium absorbed by the body. Iron status is even more affected by bioavailability factors than is calcium. Iron bioavailability depends on the diet, environment and iron status of an individual. If a person is barely consuming marginal intakes of iron (just enough to prevent deficiency symptoms), then factors negatively affecting iron bioavailability may cause that person to become iron deficient. If iron intake is borderline, a person may reduce his risk of iron deficiency by reducing factors that negatively affect bioavailability and increasing factors that increase iron bioavailability.

Heme iron and non-heme iron

A person's diet is a major factor affecting iron bioavailability. Iron is found in two forms in the diet — *heme iron* and *non-heme iron*. Heme iron is found in meats. It is iron associated with the hemoglobin and myoglobin in meat. Between 20 and 30% of heme iron is absorbed from foods. Non-heme iron is the iron found in plants, vegetables, mineral sources (with only a small amount found in animal products). Only 2 to 15% of the dietary non-heme iron is absorbed by a person. It is non-heme iron absorption that is affected by bioavailability.

Table 10-4. Factors that affect iron bioavailability.

Factor	Change in Bioavailability
1. Source of iron	Heme iron increases; non-heme iron decreases
2. Ascorbic acid	Increases
3. Dietary fibers	Decreases
4. Exercise	Increases
5. Pica	Decreases
6. Iron status	Iron deficiency increases bioavailability

Iron is found in foods in two chemical states — ferrous (Fe^{++}) and ferric (Fe^{+++}). The ferrous (Fe^{++}) state is better absorbed than the ferric (Fe^{+++}) state. Therefore, any factor that increases the conversion of iron to the ferrous state will increase its bioavailability. The *acid* in a person's stomach helps change ferric (Fe^{+++}) iron to ferrous (Fe^{++}) iron, increasing its absorption. In the elderly who often do not secrete as much acid as when they were younger, not as much dietary non-heme iron is converted to the ferrous form, causing bioavailability to be reduced. *Ascorbic acid* when consumed with a meal converts ferric iron (Fe^{+++}) to ferrous (Fe^{++}) iron. In tests where volunteers ate meals with and without added ascorbic acid, the addition of ascorbic acid to the meal increased iron absorption two times over that of the test meal without ascorbic acid.

Dietary fiber causes decreased iron bioavailability from foods. In general, fibers are complex structures with charged surfaces that bind trace elements including iron, zinc and copper. Studies have shown that persons consuming large amounts of dietary fiber absorb a lower percentage of their dietary iron. For instance, only 1-2% of the iron in spinach is absorbed. Although one does not ordinarily think of coffee and tea as high fiber foods, consumption of these products with meals will significantly reduce iron absorption from that meal. Coffee and tea have some charged, fiber-like chemicals that bind iron and make it unavailable.

Does this mean that you should avoid high-fiber foods? The answer is NO! Fiber, as discussed in Chapter 4, has important health benefits. Most high-fiber foods, especially cereals, are fair sources of iron. Even though the bioavailability is less, a significant amount of iron can still be obtained from these foods. What nutritionists do not want is for people to sprinkle purified fiber sources (oat bran, Metamucil, wheat bran, etc.) onto foods such as cereals and salads prior to eating. These purified fibers reduce the amount of iron that would be available normally from those foods.

Pica

Another factor that negatively affects iron bioavailability is the practice of *pica* in pregnant women. While pica can take many forms, it is defined as the ingestion of non-foods sources. A common example of pica is the eating of white clay from river banks during the course of a woman's pregnancy. Supposedly this practice sometimes found in the rural South will cause a strong healthy baby to be born. In fact, this practice negatively impacts the health of both the mother and her child. Clay binds to dietary or supplemental iron and other trace elements, severly decreasing their bioavailability. This occurs at a time when the mother's need for these minerals is even greater than when she is not pregnant.

Another form of pica, sometimes occurring in urban areas, is the eating of paint chips off the walls of tenement buildings. Again, factors in the paint decrease mineral bioavailability. An even more important health threat from this practice is that the chips are often from lead-based paint. This can directly affect the infant's health and development.

Another very popular form of pica, especially where clay is not available, is the eating of lumpy starch, sometimes by the boxful. While the starch itself does not decrease iron bioavailability, often the woman reduces the other foods that she needs because the starch contains so many calories. Iron intake is reduced because calories are reduced, again, at a time when the woman needs even more iron than normal.

Environmental factors that affect iron bioavailability are the *altitude* at which one lives and the amount of *exercise* one undertakes. The higher above sea level that one lives, the less oxygen is in the air. The body compensates by making more red blood cells. One way it does this is by allowing the intestine to absorb more iron so that more red blood cells can be produced. Exercise also increases a person's need for red blood cells. People that rigorously exercise have more red blood cells. One of the body's responses to exercise is to increase the amount of iron absorbed from foods.

Altitude and exercise

One last factor that affects a person's ability to absorb iron is that person's iron status. A person deficient in iron will absorb more iron from foods than a person who is not deficient. As a person's body stores of iron are depleted (indicating iron deficiency), the body tries to increase the percentage of iron absorbed from the food. However, this only allows a little more iron to be absorbed from a person's food. This increased absorption of iron will not protect a person from iron deficiency over time if his diet continues to remain very low in iron.

In summary, many children and women do not consume diets that meet their RDA for iron. They especially need to be aware of the concept of iron bioavailability so that they minimize their chances of developing anemia. While enough iron can be obtained from a well-balanced diet, a multi-vitamin and mineral supplement may be necessary to meet their needs.

Function of Iron: As previously mentioned, the main function of iron is as part of hemoglobin in the red blood cells. As red blood cells pass through the lungs, oxygen is attached to the iron of the hemoglobin. Then the red blood cells travel to other parts of the body where the oxygen is used by the cells. This process is called ***respiration***. If a person is deficient in iron, he will not have as many red blood cells as normal, and he will not be able to transport as much oxygen to his tissues. A reduced number of red blood cells in the blood is called *anemia*. People with anemia often feel *tired, sluggish, and lethargic*. That is because they have difficulty delivering enough oxygen as needed to their tissues, making it difficult for these tissues to function efficiently.

Function of iron

Because iron is necessary for red blood cells and because training increases a person's red blood cell number, athletes involved in long distance events sometimes try to artificially increase the number of red blood cells in their blood. We definitely know that performance is impaired if one is deficient in iron and thus anemic. We do not have good data to support the contention that an increased number of red blood cells will transport extra oxygen to cells during exercise. This process called *"blood doping"* is an attempt to provide the body with extra red blood cells and increase performance.

In blood doping, blood is taken from an athlete three or more months prior to a major event. The red blood cells are separated from the blood and then are frozen. The athlete's body over the next three months replaces the red cells that were removed. Then, a few days before an important event, the frozen red blood cells are thawed and reinfused into the athlete, thereby increasing the number of red blood cells normally found in that person's blood. While this may give the athlete a psychological edge, whether this practice actually increases performance is highly debatable.

Zinc

Zinc: Zinc is a trace element the importance of which is just being discovered. It functions as a *co-factor* in many enzyme systems throughout the body. It is required for *normal growth* to occur in the young. Zinc is essential for *normal wound healing*. And zinc is needed for *taste buds* to function normally.

The symptoms of a zinc deficiency include *decreased taste* and *loss of appetite*. *Decreased growth* is also characteristic of zinc deficiency, partly because of the loss of appetite and partly because zinc is needed for *long bone growth*. A major cause of *dwarfism* in the world today is due to zinc deficiency. Zinc deficiency also causes *mental retardation* in growing children. Wounds heal more slowly and recovery from injuries is slower when one is deficient in zinc.

Meeting one's RDA for zinc from the diet is even more difficult than for iron. The average diet contains only 4 mg/1000 kcals. As the RDA for zinc is *15 mg per day*, this means that one needs to consume approximately 3800 kcals per day to meet one's requirement. Again similar to iron, most foods are poor sources of zinc. With the exception of oysters (8 mg/serving), only meat is a significant source of dietary zinc (3-4 mg/serving). Beans (2 mg/serving) and cereals (0.3

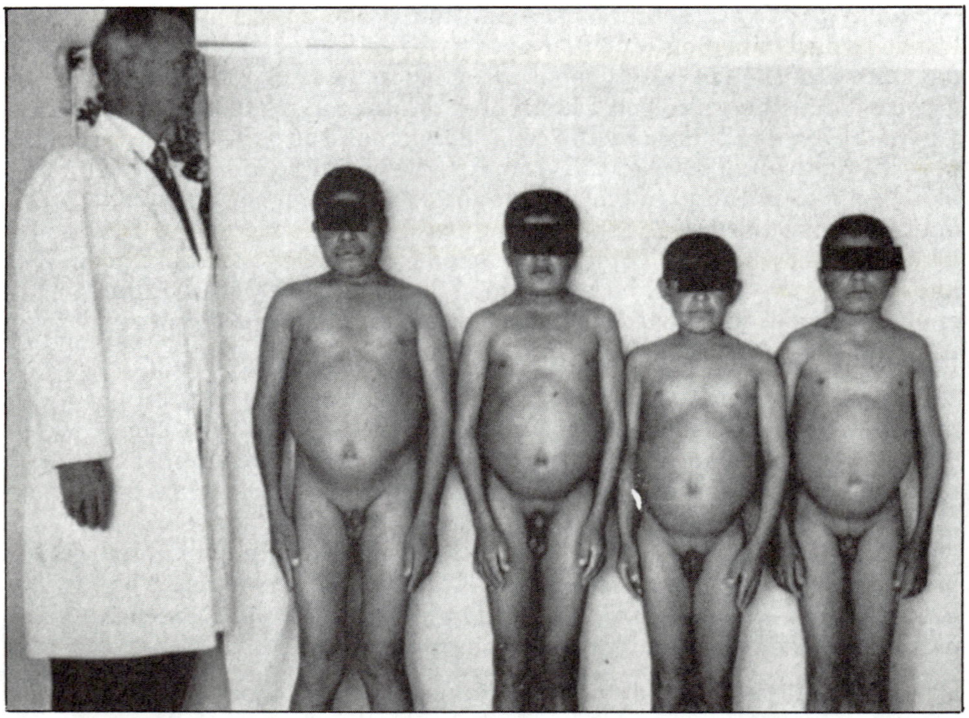

Figure 10-1. Four dwarfs from Iran. From left to right: age 21, height 4 ft, 11½ in.; age 18, height 4 ft, 8 in.; age 18, height 4 ft, 7 in.; age 21, height 4 ft, 7 in. Staff physician (left) is 6 ft in height. (From Prasad, A.S., Halsted, J.A., and Nadimi, M., *Am. J. Med.*, 31, 352, 1961.)

mg/serving), in addition to being poor sources of zinc, also have lower zinc bioavailability (because of the fiber) than meat sources. One can understand why sub-optimal intakes of zinc, especially in developing countries, are responsible for much of the dwarfism and mental retardation found there.

While most people do not eat a diet that provides optimal amounts of zinc, one should be careful about zinc supplements. Some toxicities have been associated with large, long-term intakes of zinc. These symptoms include: *fever, nausea and vomiting, anemia, loss of iron and copper stores* from the body and increased occurrence of *heart disease*. However, a multi-vitamin and mineral supplement consumed daily should not lead to zinc toxicities.

Iodine: Iodine is a trace mineral that has one specific function in the body. Iodine is necessary to produce *thyroxin*. Thyroxin is a hormone produced by the thyroid gland which is located in the neck region and controls the basal metabolic rate.

Iodine produces thyroxin which controls metabolism.

The amount of iodine in one's food is a reflection of the soil that the food is grown in. If the soil contains a lot of iodine, foods grown in that soil will be high in iodine. Conversely, foods grown in soils poor in iodine will be poor food sources of iodine. Animal sources of iodine reflect the iodine content of the foods the animal was given to eat.

A deficiency of iodine is called *goiter*. Goiter is an enlargement of the thyroid gland. It is characterized by swelling and nodule growth in the neck area. This swelling can become as large as a grapefruit on either side of the neck. What happens is that when one is deficient in iodine, the thyroid gland gets larger to try to extract more iodine out of the blood. As a person becomes more and more deficient, the thyroid gland becomes progressively larger. Once the thyroid gland reaches an enlarged state it will not shrink back to its normal size even if a person increases his iodine intake. Goiters can also be caused by substances in the foods called goitrogens. Goitrogens "tie-up" iodine from the diet, preventing its absorption. Goitrogens are found in cabbage, brussels sprouts and rutabaga. People that eat foods containing goitrogens can develop goiters even though there is enough iodine in their diet.

Goiters used to be fairly common in the United States, especially in the upper midwestern states. In the early 1900s most food was grown and consumed locally. As such, it reflected the iodine content of the local soils. In the mid-west the soil is iodine-poor. A 1920 study reported that almost one-half of the school children in Michigan had palpable (still small) but growing goiters.

"Iodized salt" has all but eliminated iodine deficiency.

Because of the endemic nature of goiter in certain areas of the country, it was decided to introduce iodine into the food supply by adding it to salt. Thus, most salt is sold as "iodized salt." This small amount of iodine in salt has been largely responsible for the elimination of goiter in the United States today. Seafoods are also very good sources of iodine. Sea salt is not a good source of iodine, contrary to some claims, because the iodine is lost when the water evaporates.

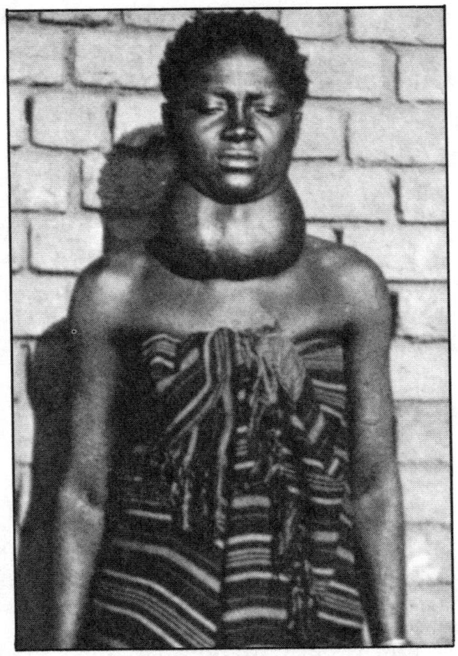

Figure 10-2. Goiter in an African woman. (From Pyke, M. *Man & Food,* McGraw-Hill Book Co., 1965.)

In summary, one needs to eat very carefully to consume his requirement for many of the trace elements. Even then it is very difficult for some segments of the American population such as women to meet their need. A multi-vitamin and mineral supplement may be warranted if one is not eating optimally. However, it should never be necessary to take more than a multi-vitamin and mineral supplement to meet one's needs.

Are you sure you're getting enough iron?

From time to time, everybody feels tired, draggy, and unproductive. There are many reasons for these downswings in energy, but for some people, the age-old claim that the cause is "iron-poor blood" may, in fact, be accurate. Worldwide, iron deficiency is considered one of the most common nutritional problems, and even in industrialized nations, including the United States, its occurrence has been estimated at 10 percent or more of the population.

Causes of iron deficiency

In most cases, iron deficiency comes from eating an iron-poor diet for long periods of time, from blood loss, or both. Recently, the Nationwide Food Consumption Survey revealed that out of more than 36,000 Americans, a third consumed less than 70 percent of the RDA for iron. Females aged 12 to 50, the years when iron intake is important to offset menstrual blood loss, took in only 59 to 65 percent. And one- to two-year-old toddlers consumed only a little more than half their RDA. The RDA does, of course, include a safety margin to meet a wide range of human needs, but intake levels of less than 70 percent trigger concern on the part of most nutritionists.

Blood loss through heavy menstrual flow, gastrointestinal disease or surgery, and too frequent blood donations can also result in iron deficiency. But the problem is seldom caused by a single factor. In a young woman, for example, deficiency may stem from a combination of low iron intake, heavy periods, repeated dieting, and too little vitamin C, which enhances iron absorption. Add to that a time of rapid growth and increased need, such as adolescence or pregnancy, and deficiency becomes inevitable without supplementation.

Although the most recent survey on iron status of people in the United States, conducted by the Federation of American Societies for Experimental Biology, showed that the over-all prevalence of iron-related problems is lower than previously thought, it targeted certain at-risk groups. Specifically, the study suggested that more than 9 percent of toddlers, 15- to 44-year-old women, and 11- to 14-year-old boys may be at risk for iron deficiency.

Types of iron in foods

Iron in foods comes in three forms. *Heme* iron is found only in animal foods: red meats, veal, pork, poultry, and seafood, but not in milk products. About 40 percent of the iron in animal or fish flesh is heme iron; of that, the body can assimilate about a third.

Nonheme iron accounts for the other 60 percent of iron in animal foods and all the iron in fruits, vegetables, dried beans, nuts, and grain products. Your body can absorb only 2 to 10 percent of this form.

Where to look for iron

The iron content listed for the following foods is an approximation of the amount obtained in a 3½-ounce portion. Keep in mind that typical serving sizes of foods vary. A 3½-ounce portion is average for meat, but an ounce is a more likely figure for bread. Don't forget about calories, either—3½ ounces of oysters provide less than 75 calories, and the same amount of peanut butter has 580 calories.

Heme iron sources

Food* *(3½-ounce portion)*	Total iron *(mg)†*
oysters, raw	6.5
beef liver, fried	5.5
clams, raw	3.0
beef, lean	2.5
sardines, canned in tomato sauce	2.5
lamb, leg	2.0
shrimp	2.0
tuna, light meat, in water or oil	1.5
chicken, dark meat	1.5
light meat	1.0
pork	1.5
haddock, breaded and fried	1.0

**Meat and poultry are cooked, lean meat only.*

†These figures are obtained from the most current USDA data and may be quite different from those previously reported because of changes in food processing and more data obtained by modern techniques.

Nonheme iron sources

Food *(3½-ounce portion)*	Total iron *(mg)†*
black strap molasses	25.0
wheat germ	9.0
apricots, dried	4.5
cashew nuts, oil-roasted	4.0
lentils or kidney beans, boiled	3.5
whole wheat, pumpernickel, or enriched white bread	3.0
prunes, dried	2.5
raisins	2.0
peanuts, oil-roasted	2.0
tofu	2.0
peanut butter	2.0
broccoli, raw	1.0
Brussels sprouts	1.0
enriched white rice, cooked	1.0
enriched spaghetti, cooked	1.0
peas, canned	1.0

From *Tufts University Diet & Nutrition Letter*, October 1985, pp. 3-6. Reprinted by permission.

Checklist on how well you are meeting your iron needs

If you want to determine whether your iron intake is adequate, you could keep track of the iron in everything you eat for a week and tally up the average number of milligrams you ingest each day. But besides being a chore, that wouldn't be very meaningful, since there are so many factors that influence the amount of nonheme and additive iron your body absorbs. Instead, why not keep tabs on steps you can take to maximize your body's use of iron? The following checklist can help.

Do you regularly consume meats? __Yes __No

If not, you might want to consider having a small amount several times a week. Not only are red meats the best source of heme iron, but animal protein facilitates nonheme iron absorption. If you're trying to cut back on fat and cholesterol, select lean cuts, remove fat, and broil them. You can also get heme iron from poultry and fish, but the amount is lower. Liver is one of the richest food sources of iron and many other nutrients, but it is also high in cholesterol.

Are fruits and vegetables among your food favorites? __Yes __No

Consuming foods rich in vitamin C—citrus fruits and juices, dark green vegetables, cauliflower, cabbage, tomatoes, cantaloupe, and strawberries—can substantially increase absorption of nonheme and additive iron. The effect is proportional to the amount of vitamin C you take in. But a glass of juice or a vitamin C supplement in the morning won't take care of iron absorption throughout the day because you need it at the same time you eat iron-rich foods. Incidentally, although spinach is quite high in iron and vitamin C, most of the iron is not available.

Do you look for enriched products when you buy processed foods? __Yes __No

Even though a single serving of most refined products doesn't have a lot of iron, enriched white bread, rolls, and crackers are the number one sources of iron in the United States, ahead of red meats. But you can't assume that all refined grain foods are enriched. For example, almost all processed flours, baking mixes, and cereals have added iron. But many snack foods, crackers, frozen breakfast foods, and breading products as well as some pasta and rice are not enriched. When selecting cereals, compare labels closely, since many of the more "natural" products are lower in iron, and fortified versions vary widely in amounts. Finally, be aware that products made from "unbleached wheat flour" are not enriched unless the label says so. The types of flour to look for on labels are enriched, whole wheat, entire wheat, or cracked wheat.

Do you ever cook in iron pans? __Yes __No

When you cook acid foods, such as tomato sauce, in an iron pan significant amounts of iron can leach from the utensil into the foods.

Do you go easy on coffee and tea? __Yes __No

Coffee can decrease iron absorption by as much as 39 percent and tea, by 87 percent, when consumed with a meal. And the effect can last for some time afterward. However, one study showed that when coffee was drunk an hour before a meal it had little effect on iron absorption. The culprit appears to be not caffeine but substances called polyphenols in the beverages. You can undo some of the adverse effects with vitamin C-rich foods; a study showed that over 50 percent more iron was absorbed from continental breakfasts containing tea or coffee when orange juice was added.

If fiber is your thing, are you careful not to go overboard? __Yes __No

Bran and phytates in high-fiber foods can interfere with iron absorption. But you're only likely to run into problems if your diet is marginal in iron and you regularly eat lots of high-fiber foods or bran supplements. Consider that whole wheat bread may have five times less iron available than white bread. But, again, you can reverse some of fiber's effects with vitamin C-rich foods.

If you use dairy products rather than meat as a protein source, are you careful to eat other iron-rich foods and good vitamin C sources? __Yes __No

Because milk products are very low in iron and egg yolks contain phosphate compounds that tie up iron, you can't count on them to meet your needs. Be certain to regularly select plant foods with iron and vitamin C and consider taking a supplement with no more than 18 mg of iron.

The third type of iron in foods, *"additive"* iron, comes in both enriched products and fortified products. Enriched foods have certain nutrients—usually iron, thiamin, niacin, and riboflavin—added in levels equivalent to those in the unprocessed versions. Fortified foods, on the other hand, contain amounts of some nutrients that are above those naturally present in foods (Presently, the two terms tend to be used interchangeably.) Unfortunately, the forms of iron used as additives, including "electrolytic" and "reduced" iron as well as iron phosphate, are generally not as available to the body as natural food iron. That's because more usable additive forms would react with other food ingredients, causing unacceptable changes in the food. For the most part, dietary factors that increase the availability of natural food iron enhance the body's use of additive iron (see Checklist).

Iron's function in the body

When you consume iron, the blood stream picks up the amount absorbed through the intestines. About 70 percent ends up in hemoglobin, a protein that releases oxygen to body cells for energy production, and 4 percent is in myoglobin, another protein that transfers oxygen to muscle cells. Some of the remaining iron is involved in important cellular chemical reactions responsible for calorie expenditure. The amount of iron that the body absorbs—and thereby uses—depends on factors other than the food source of the iron. The intestines increase or decrease absorption according to your body's need (people who are iron deficient can absorb two to three times more iron than those who have an adequate supply). And while some vitamin C-rich foods help absorption, others interfere. Estimates have it that typical American diets supply 6 milligrams of iron for every 1,000 calories eaten. Generally—given all the possibilities for variation—only about 10 percent is actually absorbed. (The rest is excreted in the stools.)

Recommended Dietary Allowance for iron

	Age	Iron
infants	0.0-0.5 years	10 milligrams
	0.5-1.0	15
children	1-3	15
	4-10	10
males	11-18	18
	19-51 +	10
females	11-50	18
	51 +	10
pregnant		30-60 mg supplement
lactating		30-60 mg supplement*

**2-3 months after delivery*

Men lose, on average, about 1 mg of iron a day but store about 1,000 mg in the bone marrow, liver, and spleen. Premenopausal women, on the other hand, have an average 1.5 mg daily deficit because of menstrual blood loss, yet they can store only about 300 mg. (Out of every 100 women, 10 to 20 are thought to have no stores.) From these figures, it's not hard to see that men can meet their 10 mg Recommended Dietary Allowance for iron more easily than women (see RDA table). Not only do adult males need less iron than females and store more, they require more calories to maintain their weight and consequently have a better chance of getting plenty of iron from food. Indeed, if every 1,000 calories worth of food provides only 6 mg of iron, a young woman would have to ingest 3,000 calories a day to get the 18 mg recommended. Most women would soon become rotund consuming that many calories.

The toll iron deficiency takes

Most people think of iron deficiency as anemia. But by the time someone truly becomes anemic, iron deficiency is advanced. There are actually several stages that precede anemia.

The first thing that happens when you don't get enough iron is that your stores are emptied. (Even though the intestines can absorb a greater proportion of the iron you eat at this point, the compensation is not enough to make up for long periods of time when iron needs are not met.) This eventually results in anemia itself—blood hemoglobin levels drop, and red blood cells become small and pale.

The symptoms of anemia usually come on slowly and can include fatigue, irritability, headaches, lack of energy, and tingling of the hands and feet. In extreme cases, a bizarre craving called pica leads people to consume dirt, clay, ice, laundry starch, and other nonfood substances. Fortunately, pica usually disappears when iron deficiency anemia is cured.

Surely anemia impairs the ability to do physical and, possibly, mental work. In one study, when anemic tea pickers were given iron supplements, they were able to pick far more leaves per day. And another study showed that anemic workers who were originally seen as lazy and unintelligent by their supervisors came to be viewed as more willing, bright, and productive after they were given iron supplements.

Feelings of weakness and fatigue, however, shouldn't trigger you to start taking iron supplements. Instead, see your physician, who can order blood tests to determine if you're anemic. If the tests show your hemoglobin and the size of your blood cells are below normal, it is possible that you're iron deficient. From there, other blood tests can be performed to determine if the cause is inadequate iron intake.

Given the fact that anemia is the endpoint of iron deficiency, you may wonder why things have to get as bad as that before the problem is diagnosed. The question becomes more pressing in light of evidence that physical performance may be impaired before anemia actually sets in. Further, several studies have shown that iron-depleted children who were not yet anemic scored better on psychological tests after taking iron supplements.

But in spite of these indications that the pre-anemic stages of iron deficiency can have an effect, Kert Sabbath, MD, a hemotologist at Brown University Medical School, believes that the implications of these studies are unclear. He says there is not yet sufficient evidence to warrant routine screening for early stages of iron deficiency in adults.

On the other hand, the Food and Drug Administration's Walter Glinnsmann, MD, at the Center for Food Safety and Applied Nutrition, thinks that the studies showing effects of preanemic stages of iron deficiency raise legitimate questions. He foresees a day when tests for the early stages become commonplace.

What to do for iron deficiency anemia

If you are found to be anemic because of iron deficiency, foods alone won't replenish your body. You're going to need iron supplements in the form of ferrous gluconate, ferrous sulfate, or ferrous fumarate, to name the most commonly prescribed forms. In order to avoid the common problem of gastrointestinal upset that can accompany supplement use, it is usually advised that you start out with one iron pill daily, gradually building up to several and spreading them throughout the day.

When you take iron tablets, don't be frightened if your bowel movements turn black. Further, some people complain of constipation, although a recent study of children on iron supplements did not confirm that as a side effect. Up to three times more iron can be absorbed if you take supplements at least one hour before rather than with meals. And try to avoid having iron with coffee or tea. Consuming vitamin C-rich foods along with iron pills is not necessary, because the vitamin appears to have little impact on absorption of supplemental iron.

People who are not anemic but who want to take an iron supplement just to play it safe are not likely to experience any ill effects if they stick with RDA levels according to Dr. Sabbath. He suggests that women with heavy menstrual periods check with their physicians about the possibility of taking supplements that contain 30 mg of elemental iron for the five days they're menstruating.

Special needs of pregnancy

Pregnant women in this country are usually given a daily supplement containing 30 to 60 mg of iron because it is next to impossible to meet the RDA with foods. And even mild anemia can lead to a host of problems, such as premature delivery. A supplement is also recommended for 2 to 3 months postpartum; even though the iron needs of breast-feeding women are about the same as before pregnancy, it is a good idea to build up stores.

Unfortunately, iron supplements pose several problems during pregnancy, aside from the usual side effects. On one count, the iron in prenatal combination vitamin/mineral supplements does not appear to be highly available; research suggests that calcium and magnesium compounds in these products interfere with iron absorption (see February '84). Hence, it may be wise to take a prenatal supplement that's low in calcium or to take an iron supplement all by itself, because the other nutrients in vitamin pills are not necessary if you eat a well-balanced diet. (Some obstetricians may also advise a folic acid supplement.) If you must take calcium supplements, iron expert James Cook, MD, of the University of Kansas Medical School, thinks it makes sense not to take them at the same time as iron. As for calcium-rich foods, Dr. Cook views them as having a relatively neutral effect on iron absorption—neither positive nor negative.

During pregnancy, it's also important to make sure your diet is rich in zinc, since high levels of supplemental iron may interfere with zinc absorption. (See March '85 for zinc sources.)

Iron overload

Iron toxicity has been reported in Africans who make heavy use of foods and beer made in iron pots, but it would be almost impossible to consume too much iron from food sources alone. Most healthy adults could probably get away with consuming food iron at levels ranging from 25 to 75 mg a day without experiencing problems. In fact, Dr. Cook states that there are isolated reports of people who have taken iron supplements for decades without having ill effects.

The real concern with iron overload is hemochromatosis, a genetic disease that causes iron to accumulate in the liver, pancreas, and heart, resulting in severe damage. Luckily, it is estimated that only one to three out of every 1000 people have the two genes that can cause hemochromatosis. But Dr. Cook believes that the one in 10 people who don't have the disease itself but carry one gene for it can get into trouble with long-term ingestion of iron supplements.

Name ______________________

Section ______________________

Date ______________________

Chapter 10

QUESTIONS FOR REVIEW

1. Name three groups of people that do not eat enough iron in their diets.

   a.

   b.

   c.

2. The major function of iron is to make ______________________ .

3. The RDA for iron for men is ________ mg/day, while the RDA for iron for women is ________ mg/day.

4. The two forms of iron that are found in the diet are ________ iron and ________ iron.

5. An iron deficiency results in ______________ (decreased number of red blood cells).

6. Most foods are/are not a good source of iron.

7. List 3 factors that increase the bioavailability of iron and 3 factors that decrease its bioavailability.

Increase	Decrease
a.	a.
b.	b.
c.	c.

8. List three functions of dietary zinc.

   a.

   b.

   c.

9. Like iron, most foods are/are not a good source of zinc.

10. Iodine is necessary to make the hormone ______________________ . A deficiency of iodine is called ______________________ .

CHAPTER 11

Nutrition through the Life Cycle

Nutrition is important to a person's health at all stages of life. A mother's nutritional status affects the course of her pregnancy and the health of her baby. Proper nutrition in infancy is important because this is a developmental stage. Nutrition during the childhood and adolescent years is important because food habits learned during this period continue throughout one's life. One's nutritional status and adult nutritional habits impact significantly on the development of degenerative diseases. The elderly have many special nutritional problems related to physiological changes associated with aging. Thus, nutrition plays a role in health and well-being throughout one's life.

Nutrition and Pregnancy

Nutrition and Pregnancy: A woman's nutritional status will significantly affect her pregnancy. During pregnancy a woman's needs for most nutrients significantly increase (Table 11-1) because she must support the fetus's growth as well as her own. When intakes are not sufficient to meet the requirements of pregnancy, often the woman draws on her own stores. For instance, before vitamin and mineral supplementation during pregnancy, a common phrase was "lose a tooth for each baby." What this meant was that the increased calcium need during pregnancy was met by drawing on the woman's bone and teeth calcium. In these cases the infant was usually normal, but the health of the mother (such as increased risk of osteoporosis) suffered. However, if the pregnant woman has inadequate levels of some nutrients (such as iron or folacin) to draw upon during her pregnancy, her poor nutritional status may negatively affect the development of the fetus, usually resulting in low birth weight.

The success of pregnancy is determined primarily by the occurrence of the following three events: *premature births, live births* and *low birth weights*. While nutrition is probably not the most important factor in any of these events, it is a mitigating factor in all of them. A birth is considered premature if the gestation period (pregnancy) is less than 37 weeks. More important than premature birth (because sometimes it is difficult to establish exactly when the pregnancy began) is the number of live births and the infant's birth weight. The United States ranks only about 15th in the world in live births. Low birth weight infants (less than 2500 grams [about 5.5 pounds]) are much more likely to die or have major illnesses than infants that weigh more than 2500 grams.

Table 11-1. Changes in requirements of selected nutrients during pregnancy.

	Non-Pregnant	Pregnant
Protein (grams)	44	74
Vitamin A (RE)	800	1000
Vitamin D (ug)	7.5	12.5
Vitamin C (mg)	60	80
Thiamin (mg)	1.1	1.6
Pyridoxine (mg)	2.0	2.6
Folacin (ug)	400	800
Calcium	800	1200
Iron	18	Needs Iron Supplement

To understand how nutrition and other factors affect the course of pregnancy, one must understand the three stages of pregnancy. The three stages of pregnancy are *implantation, embryonic development* and *fetal development.* The first stage of pregnancy, the implantation stage, occurs during the first two weeks after fertilization. Often the woman is not aware that she is pregnant during this time. Major stresses or drug or alcohol use can result in termination of pregnancy often without the woman even being aware that she was pregnant.

The second stage of pregnancy is called embryonic development. During this stage, from approximately 2 to 8 weeks of the pregnancy, the embryo develops into a fetus. This is a critical stage in the development of the embryo as it is during this time that the embryo develops most of its organ systems. During embryo development a complete digestive system, a beating heart and a complete nervous system are made. If gross nutritional deficiencies exist at this time, they can lead to congenital abnormalities (birth defects) or spontaneous abortions. However, in most cases if a woman is completely deficient of a nutrient, she most likely would not get pregnant or the pregnancy would not last past the implantation stage.

During embryonic development problems occur when a woman consumes excessive amounts of nutrients or other drugs. For instance, vitamin A given to treat acne can cause birth defects. This effect of vitamin A and its derivatives occurs during the embryonic development stage. The amount of vitamin A necessary to cause birth defects is much more than a woman could consume in her diet. However, excessive consumption of vitamin supplements or the use of some anti-acne medicines (containing vitamin A derivatives) should be avoided during the early stages of pregnancy.

FAS (fetal alcohol syndrome)

Another major cause of birth defects during embryonic development is excessive alcohol consumption. Over-consumption of alcohol during pregnancy can lead to a syndrome called *fetal alcohol syndrome (FAS).* FAS, occurring in approximately one of every 750 births, is a major public health problem in the United States today. As little as 1 ounce of alcohol per day over the course of pregnancy causes an increase in the number of low birth weight infants and an increase in the number of spontaneous abortions. Three ounces of alcohol per day, especially during embryonic development, can cause full-blown FAS. FAS is characterized by facial malformations, including a shortened forehead, a flat, flared nose and mongoloid-type eyes. A person with FAS has a greatly reduced mental capacity (intelligence) and greatly decreased motor skills (coordination). While there is debate on how much alcohol must be consumed before the health of the baby is impaired (either low birth weights or FAS), it is clear that this problem does not exist in the absence of alcohol consumption. Most physicians believe that occasionally consuming alcohol will not harm the fetus, but moderation is very important.

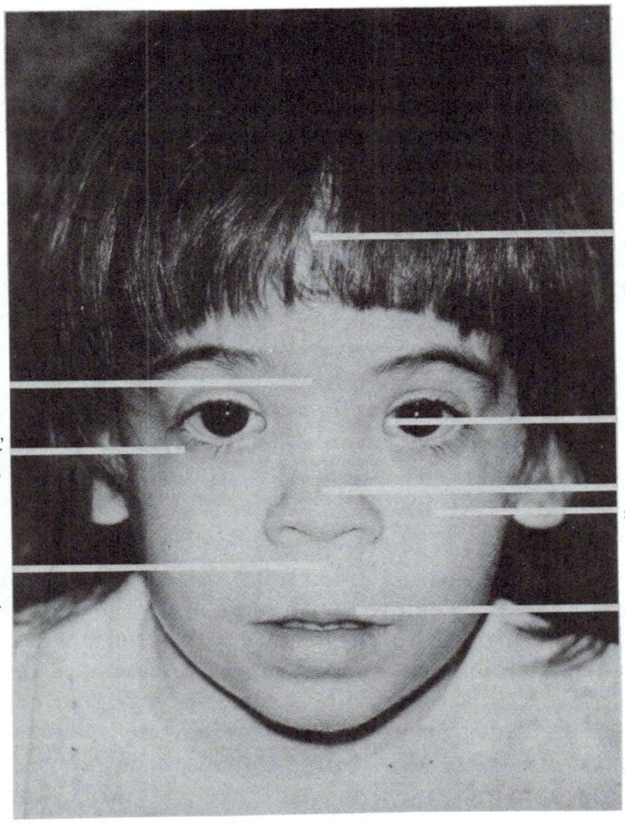

Figure 11-1. General characteristics of Fetal Alcohol Syndrome. (From Ibec, F. Fetal Alcohol Syndrome. *Nutrition Today,* Sept./Oct. 1980, Williams & Wilkens)

Pre-eclampsia affects the mother's health.

During the third stage of pregnancy (8 weeks to term), the embryo grows into a fetus. During this time malnutrition or other medical problems primarily result in a reduced birth weight or a decreased functional capacity of various tissues. Deficiencies at this time do not result in birth defects because the fetus is already formed. Among the dangers to pregnancy during this stage are excessive weight loss or weight gain. During pregnancy a woman's weight gain should be about 22-27 pounds. Pregnancy is not the time to go on a diet. There is an increased number of still-born infants and low birth weight infants in women who gain less than 20 pounds during pregnancy. Excessive weight gain during pregnancy increases the mother's risk for a condition called pre-eclampsia. Pre-eclampsia often occurs when weight gain exceeds 35-40 pounds during pregnancy. It is characterized by exceptionally high blood pressure during the last trimester of pregnancy. The high blood pressure can cause the kidneys to fail, and if not treated, cause death to the mother.

Other hazards to fetal development include *smoking, alcohol, poor diet and pica*. Smoking causes a decreased blood flow to the fetus resulting in lower birth weight infants. As previously mentioned, alcohol use increases the chance of having a low birth weight infant. If the mother is not consuming optimal amounts of nutrients, this can also cause an increase in low birth weight infants. Finally, a condition called pica can interfere with trace mineral (especially iron and zinc) absorption. Pica is the craving and eating of non-food materials during the early part of pregnancy. Pica primarily manifests itself in the South as the consumption of clay from river banks. The clay binds to trace minerals and makes them unavailable for absorption. This can lead to deficiency symptoms and health problems for both the mother and fetus. In areas where clay is not available, lumpy laundry starch is eaten, often by the boxful. While the starch does not affect mineral absorption, the consumption of so many empty calories usually means that the consumption of other foods is less. A last form of pica, occuring in urban areas, is the consumption of paint chips. These paint chips, often containing lead, are very detrimental to the health of the fetus.

One would think that since nutritionists and doctors know the increased needs associated with pregnancy, it would be possible to provide the optimal nutrition that a pregnant woman needs. Although we do know the increased needs of a pregnant woman, it is often not possible to provide a woman with the extra nutrients. Many pregnancies occur in low-income women, women who cannot afford health care. Many pregnancies occur in teenage women, many of whom have nutritional deficiencies. Many rural women are not seen by health professionals during the course of pregnancies. Many pregnant women continue to drink alcohol or take drugs during their pregnancies. Each of these factors contributes to the high infant mortality that occurs in the United States.

Although health problems in new-born infants and infant mortality in the United States is higher than health professionals would like, these numbers are improving. This is primarily due to a program called *WIC* (Women, Infant and Child Supplemental Feeding program). The WIC program has funded thousands of nutrition positions throughout the United States. Low-income women are also given pre-natal care through this program.

Nutrition and Infants: Infant nutrition revolves primarily around the question of breastfeeding, whether one breastfeeds or not. Since the mid-1960s there has been a resurgence in the number of women breastfeeding their infants. Most pediatricians feel that mothers, if they can, should breastfeed their infants. If one does not, for whatever reason, one should not feel guilty about this decision. The decision is a private one, and the advantages of breastfeeding over formula-feeding while real are generally minor.

Why should one breastfeed her infant? One answer is that breast milk is nutritionally superior to formula. The protein in breast milk is easier to digest and contains more free amino acids than formulas (which are primarily cow's-milk based). The fat content is also different; again that in breast milk is more easily digested. Mineral levels are also different in breast milk and formula. For instance, although breast milk has less iron and calcium than formula, other factors (most notably lactose) in breast milk increase the absorption of these minerals. Breast milk was designed for human infants. So far, formula manufacturers, although they are getting closer, still cannot duplicate the real product.

Breast milk also contains many factors which help the infant ward off infections. Obviously, infants born in sterile hospital environments are not as exposed to the germs one would find if the infant was born in a field. But breast milk can still provide factors that aid in establishing the right bacterial flora in the infant's intestinal tract. For instance, lactoferrin (an iron protein complex in breast milk) ties up iron so that it is not available to support the growth of pathogenic bacteria. Also, the higher lactose content of breast milk provides better food so that lactobacillus bacteria can grow; again at the expense of pathogenic bacteria. Breast-fed infants have significantly less colic than do formula-fed infants.

Some other advantages of breastfeeding over formula are:

1. Breastfeeding decreases fertility. This is especially important in third world countries as breastfeeding tends to keep the population down. As formulas are increasingly introduced in third world countries, the birth rate is increasing.
2. Breastfeeding aids in the teeth and jaw development of infants.
3. There are fewer allergic reactions in breast-fed infants.
4. There is a decrease in sudden infant death syndrome in infants that are breast-fed.
5. Breastfeeding may increase the bonding between mother and infant.

Again, it should be reiterated that whether an infant is breastfed or not is a decision each family needs to make based on their unique situation. Breastfeeding offers small advantages over formula feeding. In the United States today formula-fed infants generally thrive just as well as breast-fed infants.

Whether one breastfeeds or not, solid foods should never be introduced to an infant before six months of age. Prior to six months, an infant cannot develop the chewing and swallowing reflexes necessary to assimilate food. Also, many digestive enzymes are not available in infants until the infant is about six months of age. Thus, food is not very efficiently digested. Furthermore, the digestive tract is not completely "sealed" in infants less than six months of age. Whole proteins seem to be able to transverse the intestine in very young infants. This leads to allergic reactions to many food groups.

Nutrition and Childhood

Childhood Nutrition: During childhood a person often goes through growth spurts. Growing increases nutritional demands because it is a very energy-expensive process and because as one's size increases more nutrients are needed to function. For instance, as one grows, blood volume expands. This means that more iron is needed to make red blood cells for the extra blood. As bones grow a lot of extra calcium is needed. Another factor to be considered is that unlike the adult who has had many years to accumulate nutrients, children often do not have stores of nutrients to draw upon. Thus, with increased need and low stores it is easy to see why many children in the United States and even more around the world consume sub-optimal amounts of nutrients.

What nutrients are most lacking in the diets of children? Research has shown that many children consume iron, zinc, calcium, vitamin A and ascorbic acid (vitamin C) in inadequate amounts. In general, children in the United States eat a high-calorie, high-fat, high-sugar diet. They tend to eat foods that are not nutritionally dense. Such foods supply inadequate amounts of the nutrients listed previously. In addition food habits developed as a youngster continue into adulthood.

It is very important that children eat *a variety of foods*. It is especially important that they eat *food from each of the four food groups each day*. In fact, growing children need to eat four servings of milk and dairy products each day instead of the 2 servings needed by adults. It is only by eating a variety of foods from the basic four food groups that a parent can insure that the child is receiving a reasonable intake of all of the nutrients he needs. If a child's diet is not complete and varied, a multi-vitamin and mineral supplement may be given. In the child these should not be given more often than once every other day. Then you can be satisfied that the food the child is consuming and the vitamin supplement provide the child with all of his nutritional needs. A child should never be given more than 100% of the RDA for any vitamin or mineral in supplement form. Many of the vitamins and minerals are toxic in amounts above the requirement (as discussed in previous chapters), especially in young children.

Childhood obesity is increasing.

A major nutritional problem in the United States today is the increasing preponderance of obesity in children. Most experts believe that obesity is increasing in children today for two reasons: an *increase in accessibility of high-calorie foods* and a *decrease in activity*. Today's child is just not as active as the child of 30 or 50 years ago. In addition to decreased activity, many more processed high-fat, high-sugar, high-calorie foods are available today than ever before. Childhood obesity is much more difficult to treat than adult obesity. Besides one's body adapting to the excess fat, the food habits and sedentary lifestyle that led to the obesity are deeply ingrained in the person and very difficult to change. Remember, high-calorie foods are not inherently bad, but their consumption needs to be moderate and part of an overall diet plan. Try to substitute fresh fruits and vegetables for the snack and processed foods whenever possible.

Another food ingredient about which there is some concern in children is the consumption of sugar. Many people believe that too much sugar consumption leads to hyperactivity or aggressive behavior. While this is an attractive hypothesis, *controlled experiments have failed support this hypothesis.* Sugar provides "empty" calories and most children do not need these extra calories. The main adverse effect of sugar on the health of young people is that sugar increases dental caries (cavities).

Sugar, especially from solid, sticky sources such as caramel, increases tooth decay. The sugar gets stuck between the teeth and is used by bacteria to grow. As they grow, the bacteria produce an acid that destroys the protective enamel coating of the teeth. It is important to brush one's teeth (brushing also keeps one's gums healthy). Fluoridation (the addition of fluoride to the water supply) has greatly reduced the incidence of tooth decay in children. Fluoride works by making the enamel and tooth more resistant (or harder) to the acids of the bacteria. So the most effective protection against tooth decay is brushing, fluoridation and a reduction in sticky sugar consumption, especially between meals.

Nutrition and Adolescence

Nutrition and the Adolescent: Today's adolescent (young teen) faces many of the same problems as the child regarding nutrition. Like the child, the adolescent is growing and he has increased nutritional needs. Young people generally do not consume as much iron, calcium, vitamin A or pyridoxine as they need. Thus, it is important for the adolescent, like the child, to eat foods from the basic four food groups to try to meet his needs.

However, many more factors influence the adolescent's nutritional choices than the child's. Because of the changes occurring in them and because they exert much more control over their food choices, young people are much more susceptible to nutritional misinformation than children. Psychological changes such as puberty, the perception of his/her body and awareness of the other sex influence the adolescent's food choices. Often young people work part-time jobs which also affect the time and availability of food choices. The young athlete often receives conflicting information about foods that will affect his performance Peer pressure certainly affects diet choices. Thus, for these and probably many other reasons, it is very important that the adolescent be concerned about his food choices. If the diet is not as varied as it could be, the adolescent might take a multi-vitamin and mineral supplement to meet his/her needs. Regardless of what one hears, it is never necessary to take more than one multi-vitamin and mineral supplement per day.

Nutrition and the elderly

Nutrition and the Elderly: The elderly represent an increasing proportion of the population of the United States. Over 13% (approximately 30,000,000) of the people in the United States are over age 65. The life expectancy for a female currently age 65 is approximately 18 years, while the life expectancy for a male age 65 is about 12 years. A female currently age 75 can expect to live an additional 12 years while a male age 75 can expect to live an additional 9 years. In fact, people are living so long that there are now categories of elderly. The young elderly are those between the ages of 65 and 74 years and the aged are those over 75 years old.

As one ages, many physiological as well as psychological changes occur that affect nutritional status. Some of these changes are listed in Table 11-2. In general, the elderly need more of most nutrients because they do not absorb the nutrients as efficiently as when they were younger. Even though the elderly need more of most nutrients, their need for energy (kilocalories) is significantly less than when they were younger. The energy needed by the elderly (compared to the younger adult) is less because the elderly are not as active and the amount of lean body mass (muscle) in the elderly is much less. For instance an elderly person (age 75 years) may have only 50-60 per cent of the muscle he had when he was 30 years old. Finally, energy needs in the elderly are reduced because many of their tissue systems' functional capacities are reduced: The liver, intestine, nervous tissue and kidneys may only function at 40-50 percent of the capacity as when the person was younger. Thus, in the elderly the nutrient density of foods is very important because while they often need more nutrients they need less kilocalories.

Table 11-2. Some physiological and psychological changes of aging.

A. Physiological Changes
   1. loss of teeth
   2. decrease in taste and smell acuity
   3. decrease in stomach acid
   4. less digestive enzymes
   5. decreased absorption of some nutrients
   6. decreased kidney and liver function

B. Psychological or Sociological Changes
   1. loss of spouse
   2. living alone (single meal size)
   3. inadequate cooking facilities
   4. low income

Nutritional surveys show that the elderly are consuming less than optimal amounts of vitamin A, vitamin C, vitamin B_{12}, calcium, iron and zinc. In addition, most elderly are taking up to 8-10 different types of medication, many of which interfere with the absorption or utilization of nutrients. Given that the elderly have an increased need for nutrients, less than adequate intakes, medical problems that interfere with nutrient utilization, social problems and an expanding life span, it is clear that geriatric nutrition is becoming an increasingly important area of medicine.

What is being done to provide the elderly with the best nutrition possible? At present new RDA requirements are being developed to provide a framework for nutritional recommendations for the elderly. In addition, the government sponsors programs to help feed much of America's elderly population. Congregate feeding programs have been instituted in many cities. These programs provide one or two nutritionally complete meals per day for the elderly. In rural areas of the country or for the elderly who cannot leave their homes, a "Meals on Wheels" program has been implemented. Many times the cost of the meals is reduced or free for those elderly persons who cannot afford to pay.

In summary, nutrition is important throughout one's life. There is not any stage of life when nutrition does not affect health and well-being. Regardless of one's age, it should be clear that one should eat a diet that includes a variety of foods from the basic four food groups. Following this advice and eating foods in moderation should provide one with all of the nutrients required.

FACTS AND FALLACIES ABOUT EATING AND PREGNANCY

Now that you're eating for two . . . You shouldn't drink. Keep your weight down. Stay away from salt. Take supplements. Such are the admonitions aimed at many a pregnant woman by well-intended friends and relatives, physicians, and even local health food stores. But advice on nutritional needs during pregnancy is often contradictory, based on hearsay or out of step with current scientific knowledge, and the many commonly held myths about how to eat when a baby is on the way need to be set straight.

FALLACY You don't need all the recommended nutrients until pregnancy is under way.

FACT How a woman eats before she becomes pregnant is important not only for her health but also for her baby's. If, for example, her iron intake is marginal, she runs the risk during pregnancy of depleting her iron stores and becoming anemic. And since many women consume too little calcium throughout their lives, some experts believe that the added demands placed on calcium needs during pregnancy can increase the likelihood of osteoporosis in later years. As far as the unborn infant is concerned, it is wise for an underweight woman to try to reach a healthy weight before she becomes pregnant, because women who weigh too little when they conceive are more likely to have small babies. And the size of newborns is an important "predictor" of what their overall health will be.

FALLACY An unborn baby's nutritional needs will be met at the expense of the stores of the mother who doesn't eat well while expecting.

FACT The notion that a fetus can get all the nutrients it needs no matter what the mother eats was dispelled decades ago when women who were pregnant during World War II famines gave birth to an unusually high number of small and unhealthy babies. The effects of more subtle nutritional deficits are still not known. But an ongoing study funded by the National Institute of Child Health and Human Development is examining whether vitamin supplements taken around the time of conception will lower the incidence of certain birth defects.

FALLACY Because a pregnant woman is eating for two, she can eat twice as much.

FACT That would appear to be the case, considering that, during pregnancy, the RDA for iron nearly triples; for folic acid, it doubles; and for calcium, it increses by 50 percent (see RDA chart). However, a pregnant woman needs only about 15 percent more calories, amounting to about 150 extra calories a day during the first three months and 350 additional daily calories for the remainder of the pregnancy. But since a tuna sandwich alone could easily meet that need, those extra calories don't really amount to much additional food. As a result, a pregnant woman has to carefully choose what she eats in order to pack in the higher amounts of vitamins, minerals, and protein she requires.

FALLACY The less weight gained during pregnancy, the better.

FACT This misconception, widely held a few decades ago, was based on the belief that women who gained no more than 15 to 20 pounds would be less likely to develop complications during pregnancy and would have smaller, more easily delivered babies. Neither theory has held up over the years, however. Currently, most obstetricians believe that a weight gain of 22 to 27 pounds is acceptable. However, some research suggests that the healthiest babies are born to women who gain more than that. Marian Frank Zietlin, PhD, at Tufts University School of Nutrition, is conducting a study to see if that is so. Surely, underweight women should gain at least 30 pounds by the time they have the baby.

FALLACY If you gain the recommended amount of weight during pregnancy, you won't put on excess fat.

FACT That statement, alas, is simply not true. Fat deposits—often around the hips and thighs—are a natural part of a healthy pregnancy. Let's say a woman gains 27 pounds. Only about 7½ pounds is baby; 3 pounds come from an increase in the size of the breasts and uterus; and another 9 pounds is contributed by a combination of the placenta, amniotic fluid, extra blood volume, and other fluids. That leaves 7½ pounds, which is fat that is

From *Tufts University Diet & Nutrition Letter,* December 1985. Reprinted by permission.

believed to be a reserve for the mother who breast-feeds.

FALLACY As long as you gain the proper total amount of weight during pregnancy, it doesn't matter when you gain it.

FACT Many experts believe that the pattern of gaining weight during pregnancy is at least as important as the total amount. The goal should be a slow, steady gain, but the pattern for each woman will vary. So, for instance, if someone gains a large amount one month, she shouldn't panic and start to diet. The main thing to watch for is a sudden, unexplained jump in weight. That could be the result of fluid retention, which is a sign of toxemia and a serious problem if not treated promptly.

FALLACY Obese women should not go on a diet to lose weight before becoming pregnant.

FACT It all depends on how well-balanced the diet is. If carefully planned with the aid of a dietitian, weight loss is not a bad idea, particularly if it can be accomplished well before pregnancy. The reason is that obese women are more likely to develop hypertension, diabetes, toxemia, and urinary tract infections when they're pregnant. In addition, obese women may run a higher risk of having unhealthy babies than women of normal weight. Even when obese women have no other complications during pregnancy, they are more likely to have Caesarean deliveries than women who are not obese.

FALLACY If you are overweight, you don't have to gain weight during pregnancy because your baby can draw on your reserves.

FACT One study showed that out of a group of pregnant, overweight women, infants born to those who gained the least weight had double the death rate of babies born to mothers who had higher gains. In other words, a pregnant woman should definitely not diet, because restricting calories limits the chances of getting the right amounts of nutrients, such as calcium and protein. Strict diets also can cause the body to produce by-products of metabolized body fat that some researchers believe may affect the brain of the fetus.

A number of obstetricians strongly advise their overweight patients to follow the normal pattern of weight gain in pregnancy. Others see no harm in holding total gain to 16 pounds—but no less—because there is evidence suggesting that it is a safe course for an obese pregnant woman. That goal can be achieved by reducing the extra calories needed to an average of 200 a day over the full term of pregnancy, but it should be done with the aid of a registered dietitian.

FALLACY A woman should not exercise while she is pregnant.

FACT It is true that pregnant women with certain medical problems, such as heart disease, should not exercise vigorously. But last spring, the American College of Obstetricians and Gynecologists recommended walking, swimming, stationary cycling, and modified forms of dancing and calisthenics as ideal forms of exercise for pregnant women as long as their pulse rate does not exceed 140 beats a minute and strenuous activity is not engaged in for more than 15 minutes. They also issued detailed guidelines for doctors to advise pregnant patients. Anyone who wants to continue an ongoing fitness program should first consult with her physician.

FALLACY When you expect twins you should "double up" on everthing you eat—and gain.

FACT Although very little research has been conducted on the needs of a woman who is carrying twins, a study done at Grady Memorial Hospital in Atlanta showed that out of 137 twin pregnancies, the healthiest babies were born to mothers who gained about 41 pounds during the typical twin pregnancy time of 36 weeks. Sherri Carlton, MMSc, RD, who led the study team, believes that tall or thin women who are expecting twins should gain somewhat more than that. She also says that the need for folic acid and protein is greater for twin than single pregnancies, but the exact increment is not known.

FALLACY A prenatal multivitamin/mineral supplement is a must for all pregnant women.

FACT There is no consensus of opinion among experts on prenatal nutrition regarding the kinds of supplements a pregnant woman should take. But nearly all agree that 30 to 60 milligrams of supplemental iron daily—best taken between meals—is essential. In addition, the American College of Obstetricians and Gynecologists advises at lease 400 micrograms of supplemental folic acid a day for most pregnant women. Prenatal vitamin/mineral supplements supply adequate amounts of both nutrients, but they're expensive, and the other nutrients in them are unnecessary if a woman eats a well-balanced diet.

FALLACY Pregnant women who take a prenatal multivitamin/mineral supplement don't have to worry too much about their diets.

FACT These supplements tend to give women a sense of security when, in fact, none provides any part of the 30 extra daily grams of protein suggested during pregnancy. And their amounts of calcium don't come close to meeting the RDA. Furthermore, questions are being raised about the availability of nutrients in prenatal supplements. For example, the magnesium and calcium in them appear to interfere with the absorption of iron. Thus, pregnant women should pay close attention to the foods they eat whether or not they take a supplement.

FALLACY Taking supplements of one or another individual nutrient is not a harmful practice during pregnancy because the mother will excrete whatever she and the fetus don't need.

FACT If there's ever a time not to experiment, it's during pregnancy. Taking vitamins in amounts that are over and above the RDA (see table)—say, in doses that are 10 to 90 times the recommended amount—may seriously harm an unborn baby. Such levels of vitamin A, for example, could cause bone deformities. And consistently high doses of vitamin C could make the baby vitamin C "dependent"—that is, requiring unusually high amounts that will not be met through normal infant feeding. In short, a healthy pregnant woman should not take any nutrient in a level that exceeds the RDA.

FALLACY You can avoid gaining too much weight during pregnancy by taking calcium supplements instead of drinking milk.

Here's What You Need

Recommended Dietary Allowances
for Women Ages 23-50

Nutrient	*Nonpregnant*	*Pregnant*
protein (gms)	44	74
vitamin A (IU)	4,000	5,000
vitamin C (mg)	60	80
vitamin D (IU)	200	400
vitamin E (mg)	8	10
thiamin (mg)	1	1.4
riboflavin (mg)	1.2	1.5
niacin (mg)	13	15
vitamin B_6 (mg)	2	2.6

Nutrient	*Nonpregnant*	*Pregnant*
folic acid (mcg)	400	800
vitamin B_{12} (mcg)	3	4
calcium (mg)	800	1,200
phosphorus (mg)	800	1,200
magnesium (mg)	300	450
iron (mg)	18	*
zinc (mg)	15	20
iodine (mcg)	150	175

* *30 to 50 mg of supplemental iron is recommended.*

Here's How You Get the Most Important Nutrients

Calcium Milk products on the order of 4 servings a day are recommended. A serving is an 8-ounce glass of milk—skim, low-fat, whole, or buttermilk; 1 cup of yogurt; 1½ ounces of hard or American cheese; 2 cups of cottage cheese; 1½ cups of ice cream or ice milk; 8 ounces of tofu, stating it was made from a calcium coagulant such as calcium sulfate; 2 cups of broccoli; or 4 ounces of salmon (with soft bones).

Protein To get the 74 grams that pregnancy calls for, have 2 to 3 ounces of any of the following three or four times a day: meat, poultry, fish, or cheese. Alternates for a serving would be 2 medium eggs, ¼ cup of peanut butter, 1 to 1½ cups of cooked dried beans, peas, or lentils.

Folic acid To help meet the doubled RDA for pregnancy, try to have at least 1 or 2 daily cups of the following folic-acid rich vegetables: spinach, turnip greens, endive, dark green lettuce such as romaine, asparagus, okra, broccoli, parsnips, cauliflower, peas, Brussels sprouts, and cabbage. Fill in with several more servings of other vegetables. Don't cook them too long because folic acid is sensitive to heat.

Zinc and iron The fact that you're taking a supplement doesn't mean you should forgo good iron sources in food, partly because most are also high in zinc. Both iron and zinc are most available in animal foods, including red meats; organ meats such as liver; seafood, especially shellfish; and poultry. Whole-grain breads and cereals as well as nuts and legumes carry both minerals, too. Milk is a good source of zinc but not iron.

Vitamin C One cup of orange juice, broccoli, red or green pepper, grapefruit juice, strawberries, Brussels sprouts, cauliflower, dark greens, or 1 orange will each come close to meeting the RDA for pregnancy. Vitamin C is destroyed by heat as well as air, so cook foods a short time and keep them covered.

Vitamin B_6 There hasn't been adequate research on the vitamin B_6 content of different foods, but it is known that good sources include liver, light-meat chicken, bananas, navy beans, and walnuts. A 3-ounce serving of each provides close to 20 percent of the RDA for pregnancy. Other good sources include tuna, halibut, avocados, peanuts, beef, salmon, and dark-meat chicken.

Thiamin, niacin, and riboflavin Four daily servings of enriched or whole-grain breads, cereals, rice, crackers, or pasta will help meet the RDA for these B vitamins. Since many processed and snack foods are not enriched, be sure to check labels when shopping. Don't assume that items with unbleached wheat flour are enriched unless they say so.

FACT That's not such a good idea because the recommended 4 daily cups of fortified milk provide the RDA for calcium, meet the RDA for vitamin D, *and* give the mother-to-be the extra 30 grams of protein she needs—all for about 350 calories if the milk is skim. If a pregnant woman can't drink milk, she should ask her physician about taking a calcium supplement to make up for what she's not getting from foods. But because calcium supplements can interfere with iron absorption, it's important not to take doses of the two minerals at the same time. And when taking more than one tablet of either mineral, they should be spaced throughout the day. Further, it is best to take calcium with meals and iron in between meals.

FALLACY Pregnant women instinctively crave foods their bodies need and develop a natural aversion to things that aren't wholesome.

FACT To the contrary, even sophisticated, knowledgeable women can develop a craving for such bizarre things as clay, ashes, or laundry starch. They should try to resist such compulsions. But if they can't, they should not be reluctant to discuss the problem with their obstetricians, for it may be an overt sign of iron deficiency. Pregnant women also commonly crave foods that have nothing to do with nutritional needs. It's okay to give in to them as long as no major food groups are neglected and weight gain is acceptable. And cravings can be put to good work. If, for example, a woman craves salty snacks, she can choose salted enriched or whole-grain crackers or bread sticks. If sweets are the foods she can't resist, a glass of milk could go along with enriched cookies.

As far as aversions are concerned, many pregnant women develop a distaste for coffee and alcoholic beverages.

A dislike for vegetables that are rich in folic acid—those in the cabbage family, which includes broccoli—is fairly common, too.

FALLACY You can minimize retention of fluids by restricting your intake of salty foods.

FACT Salt used to be a no-no for pregnant women because of a belief that restricting salt intake would help prevent toxemia. But that did not prove true and is no longer advised unless the mother has a medical problem such as hypertension. Further, it is now known that pregnancy causes the body to lose more salt than normally, making dietary needs somewhat higher. When purchasing salt, pregnant women should check labels to be certain they get the iodized kind.

FALLACY A healthy pregnancy is one without discomfort.

FACT There is no question that even the healthiest of pregnancies often brings about a number of discomforts that relate to how a woman eats. Morning sickness, which actually occurs at any time of day, can be alleviated with dry crackers or toast. Another tip is to have meals without beverages, waiting until later to drink liquids. Women who have morning sickness should take advantage of times when they feel good to eat nutritious foods that they cannot stomach when nausea strikes. And if they have several small meals with snacks in between rather than a few large meals each day, the onslaughts of morning sickness will probably not be as severe. Small, rather than large, meals also help reduce heartburn, another common discomfort of pregnancy. In addition, it's a good idea to stay away from fatty or greasy foods and heavily spiced dishes as well as caffeine if heartburn is a problem. For constipation, an increase in whole-grain breads and cereals, fruits, and vegetables is recommended. Prunes and prune juice can help, too, because they contain a natural laxative. And drinking plenty of fluids and regular exercise can get the intestines moving.

FALLACY An alcoholic beverage is okay when you're pregnant as long as it's not a lot.

FACT Since no "safe" level of alcohol intake has been established for women who are expecting, abstinence is probably the best advice. However, a number of obstetricians see no harm in having an occasional dilute drink, a small glass of wine, or a beer once or twice a week. But Eileen Ouellette, MD, a pediatric neurologist at Harvard Medical School and expert on fetal alcohol problems, says a fair amount of research is now showing that as few as one to two drinks a week may have an adverse effect on an unborn child, particularly in lowering birth weight and increasing the risk of prematurity. She agrees with the Surgeon General that staying away from alcohol is the safest course for pregnancy. Alcohol intake should even be curbed when a woman is consciously trying to conceive. That doesn't mean that you should panic if you've had a few drinks before you knew you were pregnant. Being careful for the remainder of the period will help insure a healthy outcome.

FALLACY Mothers-to-be should avoid caffeine-containing beverages and foods.

FACT While caffeine has been shown to cause birth defects in newborn rats whose mothers were fed amounts equivalent to those in 18 or more daily cups of coffee, studies of people have not confirmed this link. The safest advice for heavy consumers of caffeinated coffee, tea, colas, and cocoa products is to cut back during pregnancy. But there is no evidence of any harm in having a daily cup or two of coffee. Remember, however, that both coffee and tea can markedly interfere with iron absorption, so don't wash down your supplements with them. And if you drink herbal teas as a substitute for coffee or regular tea, be careful not to go overboard—the effects of their ingredients have not been studied scientifically.

FALLACY Foods and beverages sweetened with aspartame and saccharin are taboo for pregnant women.

FACT Neither sweetener has been shown to be detrimental to pregnant women, but most experts are uncomfortable with indiscriminate use. The safest practice, once again, is moderation. Having a daily can of soda sweetened with Nutrasweet or a packet of Equal on cereal would certainly be considered reasonable use. But for the small number of women who know they cannot properly metabolize phenylalanine, an amino acid in aspartame, use of Nutrasweet and Equal should probably be eliminated.

Name ____________________

Section ____________________

Date ____________________

Chapter 11

QUESTIONS FOR REVIEW

1. A woman's nutritional status will/will not affect her pregnancy.

2. A low birth weight infant is one that weighs less than 2500 grams (about 5.5 pounds) at birth. Low birth weight infants are more/less likely to have medical problems than a normal weight infant.

3. Over-consumption of alcohol during pregnancy can cause fetal alcohol syndrome (FAS). FAS is characterized by:

   a. facial abnormalities

   b. ↓ IQ

   c. ↓ motor functions

4. Pregnancy is/is not a good time to diet as the amount of weight gained during pregnancy is/is not important.

5. A woman's weight gain during pregnancy should be about 28 - 30 pounds.

6. List four reasons why a woman should breast feed her infant.

   a. ↑ lactose

   b. protein diff

   c. fat diff (more unsaturated for breast)

   d. fertility ↓

7. Solid food should never be given to an infant before 5-6 months of age.

8. Obesity is increasing in younger children in the United States. Name two reasons why this might be occurring.

   a. T.V

   b. foods

9. Most research suggests that sugar does/does not contribute to hyperactivity in children.

10. Sugar does/does not contribute to dental caries (cavities).

11. List 4 reasons why teenagers may not eat a completely balanced diet.

a. peer press

b. athlete

c. growth

d. acne

12. The elderly need more/less nutrients than when they were younger.

13. List 4 reasons why the elderly may not consume adequate nutrients.

a. loss spouse

b. retirement

c. low income

d. no taste

CHAPTER 12

Nutrition and Performance

The effects of nutrition on athletic performance is one of the most controversial areas of nutrition. Contrary to the opinions of many, nutrition supplements cannot enhance performance above an athlete's normal capacity. The well-nourished athlete is able to perform up to his maximal capacity, whereas the malnourished athlete is not. Nutrition can only negatively affect performance; it cannot enhance it. This chapter discusses this relationship between nutrition and performance.

Water and performance

Water: Perhaps the most overlooked and important nutrient that affects performance is water. Although water has not been previously discussed, it is considered an essential nutrient. Because water is ubiquitous, we take it for granted. When one exercises, the body sweats. It is the evaporation of water from the body that cools the body and maintains body temperature. As much as one-half gallon of water can be lost from the body per hour during exercise. This water needs to be replaced or performance suffers. Only a 5 percent drop in body weight (due to water loss) will significantly decrease performance. If water is not replaced during exercise, eventually one stops sweating and body temperature rises. When this happens, heat stroke can occur. If severe enough, heat stroke can cause death.

Fortunately, water replacement during exercise is stressed much more than in the past. It was previously thought that stopping for water during sport practice showed an athlete's lack of desire to compete. Now most coaches know that water breaks should be built into practices. You cannot wait until you are thirsty to drink water because by this time your body cells are already dehydrated. A good rule of thumb when engaging in strenuous exercise is to drink water before the event, drink 8 ounces of water every 15 minutes during the event and drink water after the event.

In most cases it is only necessary to replenish the water that your body loses. Although some salt and other nutrients (most notably potassium) are lost in sweat, it is more important to replace the water. Most people's diets contain enough salt to replace that lost during exercise. As one becomes acclimated to exercise, fewer minerals are lost in sweat. A replacement fluid sports drink such as "Gatorade," while not usually necessary, could be consumed. However, these drinks should be diluted with water for the most effective re-hydration. At no time should you consume salt tablets. Salt tablets actually draw water from the cells into the intestine to dilute the concentrated salt. Salt tablets actually increase dehydration.

Macronutrients and Performance: The key macronutrient affecting long-term aerobic exercise performance is carbohydrate. You need carbohydrate (glucose stored in your muscles as glycogen) to exercise effectively for a long time. Although muscles use primarily fatty acids for fuels during aerobic exercise (long-distance, endurance exercise), some glycogen is also used. Research has shown that subjects who eat a low-carbohydrate diet for a few days are not able to work (exercise) as long as subjects eating a mixed diet or a high-carbohydrate diet. Most casual athletes do not exercise long enough for muscle glycogen to be limiting.

Carbohydrates and performance

Muscle glycogen levels can be increased prior to an athletic event by a process called glycogen loading (discussed in Chapter 4). By eating a very high carbohydrate diet (70 percent of the diet kilocalories as carbohydrates) for a few days before the event, one can increase the amount of glucose stored in the muscle as glycogen. The greater glycogen stores allow one to compete harder and longer than a person with less stores. This is the reason for the spaghetti dinners the day before marathon races. Again it must be noted that for most weekend athletes glycogen stores are rarely the limiting factor in performance.

Dietary fat and protein affect athletic performance much less. While fat is the preferred fuel for aerobically exercising muscles, dietary fat is never a limiting factor in performance. And as most Americans consume dietary protein well in excess of their needs, it also does not affect performance.

The pre-event meal

One factor that does affect performance is the *pre-event meal.* This meal should be eaten no later than 4-5 hours before an event. Eating closer to an event causes blood to be shunted from the muscles to the intestine. In addition to making one feel sluggish, this can significantly decrease blood flow to the muscle and impede performance. The meal should be light and not contain too much fat. Fat slows down the digestive process. The meal should contain some protein but primarily complex carbohydrates.

Sugar is to be avoided as much as possible during an athletic event. First, concentrated sources of sugar cause water to be moved into the intestine to dilute the sugar. This can increase the rate of dehydration during an event. Second, sugar is very quickly absorbed into the body causing metabolic changes that do not enhance performance. Many people believe that sugar will increase blood glucose levels (which tend to fall during long distance events). In fact, high intakes of concentrated sugar will have the opposite effect, eventually causing blood glucose levels to fall even further.

Vitamins and minerals

Vitamins and Minerals: Vitamins and minerals only affect performance in a negative manner. If you have less than optimal level intake of a vitamin or mineral, your performance will suffer. A vitamin or mineral deficiency means that your body does not have all the "machinery" present to allow one to perform to his maximal capacity. For instance, if one is not consuming enough iron, one will not be able to make as many red blood cells as normal. Too few red blood cells means that one is unable to carry as much oxygen as needed during exercise. As a result one cannot perform up to maximum capacity.

While a deficiency of a vitamin or a mineral will negatively affect performance, excessive consumption will not enhance performance. Taking extra vitamins or minerals will not increase one's exercise capacity above normal. Consuming extra iron will not cause more red blood cells to be made. This is also true of other vitamins and minerals; taking extras will not enhance performance.

It is true that intensive training will slightly increase one's need for some vitamins and minerals (perhaps by 10-20 percent). Sometimes this modest increase in need is used as a selling tactic. Vitamin and mineral retailers often suggest that because one is exercising his needs for vitamins are much greater than normal. Again, this is just not true. Most of the time one's slight extra needs can be met by the diet. If one is worried that his diet is not supplying enough vitamins and minerals, a multi-vitamin and mineral tablet could be taken. You do not need to take any higher doses than this!

Ergogenic aids

Ergogenic Aids: Ergogenic aids are supplements that supposedly enhance performance. Many substances are sold as ergogenic aids, including caffeine, many vitamins, bee pollen and carnitine. In controlled testing of many of these substances, an ergogenic effect is not found. Besides costing money, readily available ergogenic aids generally provide only a psychological effect. This is, if you think you will do better, most of the time you will. People, especially athletes, are always looking for an advantage. Sometimes a pill will help just because a person thinks it will help. About the best you can hope for with most ergogenic aids is that they will provide some psychological aid and not cause any physical harm.

Bee pollen

Bee pollen is an example of an ergogenic aid that, besides not enhancing exercise performance, actually can cause physical harm. Bee pollen has been sold for many years as a supplement to stimulate endurance. In controlled, double-blind laboratory experiments no effect of bee pollen was found on exercise performance. But it is well-documented by over hundreds of cases, including some deaths, that the ingestion of bee pollen causes allergic reactions in some people. People who are allergic to bee stings can also be allergic to bee pollen.

Most ergogenic aids that have been carefully tested have failed to enhance performance. Fortunately, most do not have the major toxic side-effects of bee pollen. Remember, there really are no shortcuts to maximal performance especially for the elite athlete. First, you must have the genetic capabilities to excel at your sport. If you have the wrong muscle structure for long distance running, you will never be able to run long distances very fast. You will never be able to compete with those more genetically blessed. Second, to succeed in your area you must train. Ergogenic aids are not a shortcut to training. All the ergogenic aids in the world will never allow an untrained athlete to beat a trained athlete. And for most weekend athletes, even if ergogenic aids did make a small difference in performance, what would be the point? The weekend athlete should only compete against himself, being the best that he can be.

Another category of suggested dietary aids are those that increase one's muscle building capacity. These include extra dietary protein, extra pyridoxine (B_6), extra amino acids (especially lysine, arginine and ornithine) and dibencozide. Extra protein and pyridoxine supposedly build muscle faster in weightlifters. Large intakes of pyridoxine, besides being ineffective in accelerating muscle building, have been found to cause nerve deterioration (including paralysis). Extra consumption of the amino acids lysine, arginine, and ornithine supposedly cause the body to produce more growth hormone. Growth hormone is a hormone that affects one's body composition (the amount of muscle and fat), but there is little evidence that one can control its production through the diet. Dibencozide is a dietary aid that health food stores are selling as a supplement that accelerates muscle growth. This is currently a very popular supplement because its name sounds like a steroid. Dibencozide is a common derivative of vitamin B_{12} and has no known effects on muscle metabolism. Just as in training for an endurance event, there are no shortcuts to building one's physique. Only hard work and lifting weights can make muscles, not supplements.

In summary, malnutrition can only hurt performance. An athlete who competes while lacking water or other nutrients cannot perform to his maximal potential. If one is eating a well-balanced diet with foods from all of the basic four food groups, it is possible to consume all of the nutrients needed. If in doubt, then a multi-vitamin and mineral supplement could be taken (especially by women). There are no advantages to consuming extra vitamin or mineral supplements. Also, ergogenic aids are generally ineffective in enhancing performance, are expensive and sometimes cause toxic side effects.

Vitamins and Minerals as Ergogenic Aids

Virginia Aronson, MS, RD

Ms Aronson is author of *30 Days to Better Nutrition* and a former nutritionist with the Harvard School of Public Health in Cambridge, Massachusetts. Ralph A. Nelson, MD, PhD, editor of Nutrition and Fitness, is director of research and professor of nutrition at the Carle Foundation in Urbana, Illinois.

Nutrition articles and advertisements in popular sports magazines have convinced naive consumers that active individuals require large doses of nutritional supplements. The supplement business has blossomed into a multibillion-dollar industry because of large-scale consumption of these products. Of the adult population, both active and sedentary, 40% to 50% rely on self-prescribed vitamin supplements,[1] and athletes, coaches, and athletic trainers are choice targets for the supplement sales force.

Athletes must stay on guard against false promises. Clearly, it is not possible to change average athletes into champions simply by altering their diet. Nutrient supplements require careful consideration, not only because of possible ergogenic effects but because of the potential health consequences of overzealous supplementation.

Effective Ergogenic Aids

"Ergogenic" refers to anything that helps increase work performance, either by directly benefiting the body's physiological capacity or by removing physiological restraints. Ergogenic aids include mechanical, psychological, physiological, pharmacological, and nutritional aids. The nutritional aids are probably most abused by athletes.[2]

Ergogenic properties have been ascribed to nearly every nutrient and to a wide array of pseudonutritional substances. However, diet manipulation has improved sports performance in only a few documented cases. For example, studies in the 1960s confirmed the importance of carbohydrates for endurance athletes; however, carbohydrate loading techniques have changed since that time, and the effect on glycogen stores is not clear. And while water may be an excellent nutritional supplement (hyperhydration before competition can aid performance in endurance events by preventing dehydration and elevated body temperature), water intoxication is always a danger; it can even lead to comatose states. Caffeine may be ergogenic, but only in endurance

From *The Physician and Sport Medicine*, March 1986, pp. 209-212. Copyright, 1986, by McGraw-Hill Publishers.

Table 1. Uses and Abuses of Vitamins

	Exercise-Related Functions	Advertising Claims for Athletes	Side Effects and Toxicities
Vitamin B Complex		Increases energy and endurance, enhances performance, delays fatigue	
Thiamine	Carbohydrate metabolism, nervous system function		Interferes with absorption of other B vitamins
Riboflavin	Cellular energy release and respiration		Relatively nontoxic
Niacin	Cellular energy processes and respiration, carbohydrate metabolism, and fat synthesis		Flushing, itchy skin, headache, diarrhea, nausea, low blood pressure, fainting, irregular heartbeat, liver damage
Pyridoxine (B_6)	Amino acid and protein metabolism, RBC formation		Liver damage, nerve damage (sensory ataxia), limb impairment of vibration sense
Folacin	Regulation of tissue processes, RBC formation		Gastric upset; sleep disturbances, malaise, irritability; masks certain anemias
Biotin	Synthesis of glycogen and fat, amino acid metabolism		Depresses secretion of gastric hydrocholoric acid
Pantothenic acid	Energy and tissue metabolism		Diarrhea, water retention
B_{12}	Maintenance of nerve tissue, RBC development		Liver damage, some allergic reactions
Vitamin C	Tissue maintenance and repair, resistance to infection	Protects against illness and infection, aids in rapid recovery from injury	Gastrointestinal upset, increases need for vitamin E, interferes with copper and iron status, may cause kidney stones and gout, interferes with pregnancy
Vitamin E	Maintenance of cell integrity, muscle metabolism	Improves performance, increases endurance	Depression, fatigue; flu-like symptoms; interferes with vitamins A and K; hypertension, phlebitis, clots; gynecomastia
Vitamin A	Maintenance of proper vision, resistance to infection	Improves vision and immunity to infection	Anorexia, hair loss, increases cranial pressure, hypercalcemia, bone and kidney damage, liver damage, birth defects
Vitamin D	Normal bone growth and development	Builds stronger bones	Anorexia; weakness; hypercalcemia; deposits in soft tissue; irreversible kidney damage; damage to heart, lungs, and tissues surrounding joints
Vitamin K	Normal blood clotting	Aids in recovery from injury	Interferes with normal clotting; liver damage

Table 2. Uses and Abuses of Minerals

	Exercise-Related Functions	Advertising Claims for Athletes	Side Effects and Toxicities
Sodium, potassium	Maintenance of normal fluid balance, regulation of body systems including heartbeat and hydration	Sweat loss necessitates supplementation	Salt tablets irritate the gastrointestinal tract, cause dehydration and cramps
Chromium	Normal blood sugar metabolism	Aids carbohydrate metabolism to delay fatigue	Liver and kidney damage
Selenium	Protection of tissues against oxidative damage	Delays fatigue	Hair loss, brittle nails, skin lesions; fatigue; can be fatal in acute poisonings
Zinc	Protein synthesis and tissue repair	Speeds wound healing, losses incurred with exercise necessitate supplementation	Anorexia; nausea; diarrhea; lethargy; dizziness; muscle pain; interferes with copper metabolism, calcium and iron absorption; may impair immune response, decrease blood levels of high-density lipoproteins, trigger bleeding of ulcers
Iron	Oxygen transport to tissues for energy	Reduces fatigue, weakness; improves performance, endurance; supplementation required by all athletes	Overdoses have caused death in children; dangerous for adults with hemochromatosis

events lasting longer than two hours.

Vitality Through Vitamins?

Despite the controversial reputation of nutritional ergogenic aids, little confusion exists among researchers. Current recommendations are clear and simple: A normal varied diet with adequate fluid intake and enough food to meet elevated calorie requirements can also meet vitamin and mineral requirements if foods are selected wisely and carbohydrates are emphasized as the major calorie source.

Surveys show that three of four adults believe that taking extra vitamins will provide additional energy, no matter how adequate the diet.[3] Most people consider vitamins to be intrinsically safe, yet each year thousands of cases of vitamin poisoning are reported.[4] There are also numerous unreported cases of ill effects caused by naive abuse of vitamin supplements. A survey in seven Western states found that more than 8%, 11%, and 16% of those questioned were consuming potentially toxic amounts of vitamins A, C, and E, respectively.[5]

Ergogenic properties have been ascribed to vitamin C, vitamin E, and the various B complex vitamins. Studies have shown that vitamin supplements help sports performance only if nutrient deficiencies exist. In short, vitamins are incapable of enhancing performance.[6-9] More extensive research will be needed to answer the questions of whether and how athletic training alters the body's vitamin requirements. Meanwhile, "athletic paks" of vitamin supplements are sold along with unproven claims to those seeking a competitive edge. The uses and abuses of vitamins are described in table 1.

Vitamin B Complex

One popular supplement that athletes consume is the vitamin B complex. There are eight B vitamins—thiamine, riboflavin, niacin, pyridoxine, folacin, pantothenic acid, biotin, and B_{12}—that work together to ensure proper digestion, muscle contraction, and energy release from body stores. Since the B vitamin complex is water soluble, there is little body storage. However, large intakes of certain B vitamins may cause side effects. Thus, it is unfortunate that advertisements push excessive doses of B supplements.

Studies evaluating the effect of B supplements on performance fail to support their use.[2] Diet requirements for thiamine can be easily met with high carbohydrate foods even though high-level endurance activities elevate thiamine requirements. And though one recent study shows that extra riboflavin may be needed in the diets of active women,[10] food alone can provide that amount. Niacin in large doses might actually block release of free fatty acids and speed up use of muscle glycogen.[2] Pyridoxine and folacin can be depleted by alcohol intake, use of oral contraceptives, or high protein diets, but these supplements have not been shown to enhance performance.

A deficiency of vitamin B_{12} can lead to anemia and impair endurance activities, but a deficiency is unlikely because most people can store this vitamin for two to three years. Despite the popularity of precompetition shots of B_{12}, their usefulness in the absence of a diagnosed deficiency has not been demonstrated.

Vitamins C and E

Since deficiencies in vitamin C or vitamin E are not common in the United States, it is surprising that these are currently the two most popular vitamin supplements. Vitamin C helps maintain body tissues including cartilage and bone, helps heal wounds, aids in iron absorption, and is required for the formation of certain hormones excreted during stressful situations such as heavy exercise. Like the B complex, vitamin C is soluble in water, so excesses are excreted. No studies support the efficacy of vitamin C supplementation as an ergogenic aid, and undesirable side effects have been noted with large doses.

Vitamin E may also pose problems when taken in excess.[11] Furthermore, no performance benefits have been demonstrated in humans who use vitamin E supplements.[12-14] But a deficiency can cause abnormal muscle function in animals and decrease tolerance to periods of hypoxia.

Vitamins A and D are less popular with athletes, but they are far more toxic when taken in megadoses. Vitamin K is not often promoted tc athletes.

Minerals as Ergogenic Aids

Although not as popular as vitamins, certain minerals are also advertised as endurance enhancers. But the need for electrolyte replacement is often exaggerated, as is the need for supplementing chromium, selenium, and zinc. However, research is still being conducted to establish the actual effects of training on the body's mineral requirements. In the meantime, athletes are vulnerable to unsupported claims about minerals and need to be warned about potentially toxic side effects (table 2).

Mineral losses are incurred while sweating profusely during strenuous exercise, especially in hot weather. Although sodium depletion is a common concern among athletes, the average American consumes at least ten times the amount required to replenish daily losses.[15] Training should include environmental adaptation so that proportionately more sodium and other electrolytes can be retained and more fluids lost during exercise. Electrolyte supplements are unnecessary for the well-trained, well-fed athlete.

Chromium is an essential mineral whose metabolically active form, glucose tolerance factor (GTF), is required for maintaining normal glucose metabolism. Chromium metabolism is not yet fully understood, but since GTF plays a role in carbohydrate metabolism, GTF supplements are claimed to enhance endurance and aid sports performance. Unfortunately, certain forms of GTF are toxic and have resulted in renal damage.[16]

Toxic states are also easily reached with selenium. It functions with vitamin E to help protect cells from oxidative damage. But no evidence exists to indicate a deficiency in US residents.[17]

Zinc acts as a cofactor for regulating the activity of specific enzymes involved in nutrient metabolism, but there is no evidence that zinc supplements offer benefits to healthy people with adequate dietary intakes. Prolonged intake of zinc supplements can result in serious side effects, including reduction in high-density lipoprotein cholesterol levels.[18] These levels are elevated with exercise and are believed to protect against heart disease.

On the other hand, iron supplements may be appropriate for certain athletes with a documented deficiency. Adolescent males and females of childbearing age are especially susceptible to iron-deficiency anemia because of growth demands or menstrual losses. In addition, the metabolic consequences of endurance exercise appear to have a depleting effect on iron status.[19] Thus, athletes need to monitor iron intake, especially if they belong to one of the above groups or if they consume low iron diets (vegetarians) or low calorie diets (weight watchers).

Unrealistic Expectations

Individuals vary widely in response to nutrient supplementation depending on their age, body weight, metabolism, diet, and nutrition and health status. In some people, toxicities can result with as little as ten times the Recommended Daily Allowance of a particular vitamin or mineral, while others can tolerate excessive doses with little visible effect. Perhaps the real threat to athletes from abuse of supplementation is the unrealistic expectation that it will aid performance—leading them to ignore the importance of a balanced diet, adequate rest, and proper training.

The increased energy expenditure of athletes requires additional calories, especially from carbohydrates, plus plenty of fluids. These increased nutritional needs can easily be met by including generous servings of wisely selected foods. As long as an athlete's diet is well balanced, there is no documented need for extra vitamins and/or minerals. Unless a specific deficiency is diagnosed by acceptable medical methods, athletes and their coaches are wise to avoid the temptation to use nutritional supplements.

References

1. Trost J: Consumer nutrition attitudes and behavior: current vitamin usage data, in Vitamin Supplementation: A Factual Perspective. Nutley, NJ, Hoffman-LaRoche, 1983, pp 62-70
2. Williams M: Nutrition for Fitness and Sport. Dubuque, IA, Wm C Brown Co, 1983
3. US Dept of Health, Education and Welfare: Consumer Nutrition Knowledge Survey. Washington, DC, FDA Bureau of Foods, 1974
4. Harar J: Myths of vitamins. FDA Consumer 1974;8:4-9

Name ______________________

Section ______________________

Date ______________________

Chapter 12
QUESTIONS FOR REVIEW

1. Nutritional supplements can/cannot enhance an athlete's performance above normal.

2. __Water__ is the most important nutrient in strenuous exercise.

3. Salt tablets are/are not recommended when undertaking heavy exercise.

4. The pre-game or performance meal should be eaten no later than how many hours before the event? __4-5__ This meal should be low in dietary __fat__ but high in dietary __complex carbohydrates__ .

5. Sugar is a good/poor source of energy during long-term exercise.

6. A vitamin or mineral deficiency will __negate__ performance, but taking extra vitamins or minerals will not __help__ performance.

7. Supplements that supposedly increase physical performance are called __ergogenic__ __aids__.